HYPERFITNESS

HYPERFITNESS

12 WEEKS TO CONQUERING
YOUR INNER EVEREST
AND GETTING INTO
THE BEST SHAPE
OF YOUR
LIFE

▲

Sean Burch

AVERY
A MEMBER OF PENGUIN GROUP (USA) INC.
NEW YORK

AVERY

Published by the Penguin Group

Penguin Group (USA) Inc., 375 Hudson Street, New York, New York 10014, USA • Penguin Group
(Canada), 90 Eglinton Avenue East, Suite 700, Toronto, Ontario M4P 2Y3, Canada (a division of Pearson
Canada Inc.) • Penguin Books Ltd, 80 Strand, London WC2R 0RL, England • Penguin Ireland,
25 St Stephen's Green, Dublin 2, Ireland (a division of Penguin Books Ltd) • Penguin Group (Australia),
250 Camberwell Road, Camberwell, Victoria 3124, Australia (a division of Pearson Australia Group Pty Ltd)
Penguin Books India Pvt Ltd, 11 Community Centre, Panchsheel Park, New Delhi–110 017, India •
Penguin Group (NZ), 67 Apollo Drive, Rosedale, North Shore 0632, New Zealand (a division
of Pearson New Zealand Ltd) • Penguin Books (South Africa) (Pty) Ltd, 24 Sturdee Avenue,
Rosebank, Johannesburg 2196, South Africa

Penguin Books Ltd, Registered Offices: 80 Strand, London WC2R 0RL, England

First trade paperback edition 2008
Copyright © 2007 by Sean Burch
Photographs copyright © 2007 by Imamyar Hasanov

Most Avery books are available at special quantity discounts for bulk purchase for sales promotions, premiums,
fund-raising, and educational needs. Special books or book excerpts also can be created to fit specific needs.
For details, write Penguin Group (USA) Inc. Special Markets, 375 Hudson Street, New York, NY 10014.

The Library of Congress catalogued the hardcover as follows:

Burch, Sean.
Hyperfitness : 12 weeks to conquering your inner Everest and getting into the best shape of your life / Sean Burch.
p.   cm.
ISBN 978-1-58333-269-6
1. Physical fitness.   2. Exercise.   3. Muscle strength.   4. Health.   I. Title.
GV481.B82   2007   2007000570
613.7—dc22

(Paperback edition) ISBN-13: 978-1-58333-299-3; ISBN-10: 1-58333-299-5

Printed in the United States of America
1   3   5   7   9   10   8   6   4   2

BOOK DESIGN BY TANYA MAIBORODA

ACKNOWLEDGMENTS

The lifetime I've spent developing as a human being I hope you'll see expressed earnestly through the words and exercises in this book. My aspiration is to help all people improve their lives, better the lives of those around them, and bring their dream goals to fruition. There are so many individuals who have guided me along the trail in life, and who believed in me. For all of you (there are too many to list), I will never forget your support!

To my wife and son, who make life a sincere adventure every day, my love for you will forever remain boundless. I am in awe of you both. To my parents, for providing love, support, and nurturing. To Pam and Arthur, for providing the same to my parents.

Special thanks to Jennifer Gates—your support and guidance have been invaluable. I am particularly grateful to Tim Friend for seeing the real deal. Ethan Boldt, your assistance has been tremendous and will always be immensely appreciated. Many thanks to Megan Newman, Lucia Watson, and the rest of the sophisticated women at Avery for their valuable assistance and belief. And to all my students who have put forth the desire and the sweat—thank you for sharing your energy with me.

For providing motivation, assistance, encouragement, and an everlasting spirit: the Schou clan, Ricci family, McCabe family, James family, the White family, George Chastain, Chung Berenson, Bill Milano, Mark O'Brien, Krystal Crumpler, Marianne Ramey, Don Griner, Mike Spiller, Andy Smith, Pearl Burch, Peter Toth, Dirck Schou, Lesley Alderman, Marie and Paul Miller, Nancy and Ryan Hannigan, Charlie Patten Jr., Dallas Wolfe, Bob Becker, Bryan Geschwill, Erin Baker and Richard Owen, all at Guayakí, Judy Chambers, Susie Pfefferkorn, my sisters—Eli-Anne and Helene—and Imamyar Hasanov. To my past climbing partners—your knowledge and camaraderie were priceless.

Thanks to Bruce Lee for being light-years ahead of his time. To all the martial artists whom I've studied with—thank you for the education and wisdom. Love and laughter to my godchildren: Bella, Caroline, Chloe, Cooper, and William. And last, to those who want to make your dreams and goals a reality, I hope this book will serve you well throughout each second of your remaining days on earth.

For my son, Hans

We were high in the mountains—snow and then in the open, and soon after roaring through tunnels and over gorges. I seemed satisfied with the fact that there was no daylight. I was not in the mood for the coldness of reality and much preferred the uncertainty which the grey darkness offered.

—HANS SCHOU, SEPTEMBER 25, 1936

CONTENTS

A GRANDFATHER'S LAST WORDS

FOR TEN YEARS I HAD BEEN FASCINATED by the idea of climbing a mountain that was as high as jetliners fly. I admired high-altitude mountaineers for their boldness and sense of adventure in the face of real danger. After all, in many ways mountaineering contains all the elements in life that make one feel alive: goal setting, facing and conquering fear, enduring hardship, tasting heroism—and experiencing Mother Nature at her sweetest and most terrifying. I devoured one book after another about mountaineering, noting that a majority of them focused on the big one: Mount Everest, which at 29,035 feet is the highest peak in the world. There couldn't be a mountain more beautiful, more majestic, or more daunting.

It wasn't until 1953 that someone reached the summit and lived to tell about it, and only a handful have made the entire climb without taking any supplemental oxygen (the first two, Reinhold Messner and Peter Habeler, did so in 1978). The more I read, the more I dreamed about conquering it, unguided, and without the oxygen assist.

But, like so many people who have a daydream but leave it at that, I continued to squander my time at a job that I had neither energy nor passion for. I succumbed to the doubting going on inside and outside my brain.

Who was I to think I could climb to the highest point on earth? I had lived my entire life on the East Coast, at sea level, had no previous mountaineering experience, had no clue how to get started with such a huge endeavor, had no one who was willing to come with me (because I was so clueless at the time, who could blame them?), and had no money for the climb (climbing Everest's south side from Nepal, unguided, costs about $40,000; guided expeditions begin at $65,000. I didn't have the stomach, the heart, or even the know-how to live this dream.

I was not afraid to die on Everest; instead, I was afraid to really live. I had some goals, but they were pretty standard, generic ones. At that time, it was really only about money in the bank, a big house full of toys, and the white picket fence; I figured that at some point, I'd find a nice wife, and we'd have nice children.

At the time, I was a consultant for a company that resolves disputes for big contractors all around the globe. I was making good money, I had my own house, and I had good friends. Hey, I had met some of my so-called goals, so I should have been happy, right?

Instead, I felt unsettled. My labors were only making rich companies richer, and I knew I was doing nothing that spoke to my heart or soul. I was lonely and depressed. I found only a fleeting happiness from my mountaineering books and during my martial arts training. I'd drink beer and vodka to soothe myself. Of course, when I'd wake up the next day, I'd feel worse, a few steps further away from my Everest goal. Year after year, I'd blow out candles with birthday wishes that didn't have a prayer of coming true because I didn't put anything behind them except a heavy dose of hot air.

Then something happened: my grandfather got sick, as in terminally sick. My grandfather, Hans Schou, was the one person on earth whom I most wanted to be like. He was a world traveler, served admirably in World War II in the Pacific, spoke three languages, was a wonderful athlete and incredibly intelligent, and always seemed to have a smile on his face. I also loved him a ton, and he loved me the same. He had a lot more to teach me, because God knows I had a lot more to learn. But now my mentor of mentors was dying.

In November 1998, I visited my grandfather for the last time before he passed away. This tall, athletic, proud Norwegian-American now had tubes coming out of his nose to help him breathe, was losing weight no matter what he ate, and knew that his time on earth was coming to a close.

Fortunately, his intellect continued to burn brightly until the end. On my last visit with him, he painstakingly took the time to orally transcribe his Norwegian family history into a tape recorder for me so I could make sure future generations would know our whole family ancestry. Because he would get tired quickly, he could only speak for a few minutes at a time, but I certainly never got tired of waiting for the great tales and lessons to come out of his mouth.

I tried to soak in every word he said and, when it finally came time to go, I moved in to give him a hug and kiss good-bye. He reached and grabbed my hand, tugging me in close to his face. "Live your life, Sean. It's too late for me, but it's not too late for you," he said softly. I smiled and kissed him on the head, saying, "I will, Grandpa." Clearly he hadn't gotten his message across, for he refused to let go of my hand and peered deeply into my eyes with the most serious look I'd ever seen on his face.

Suddenly, with a burst of strength, he squeezed my hand and his voice boomed forward. "Sean! You need to live your life! There are so many things I wish I could have done but now can never do."

I was shocked to hear this from a man who I'd thought had done it all and done it well. "Grandpa, how can you say this?" I asked. "You have done so much. You've traveled the world, and have been on every variety of adventure in every corner of the earth. Grandpa, you downhill skied at age eighty-six. How many people can say that?"

He shook his head gently, as if I still wasn't getting the point. I wasn't, of course. His voice now fading, he wanted to tell me one last thing before I went. "No, Sean. I have so many dreams that are going to be left as that. Look at me. I am a shell of a man who can't even go outside for a walk. Don't let your dreams go unfulfilled. It's too late for me, but it's not too late for you. Live your life every single day on this earth, because it will be over sooner than you realize," he said.

He released his grasp and put his head back on his lounge chair. I looked at him and nodded, then squeezed his hand one last time. I said good-bye to my grandmother and by the time I turned back to Grandpa he was falling asleep. Already I was repeating his words in my head: *Live your life.* At that point in time, I thought I was. I had a well-paying job, a house, and a Norwegian model girlfriend. I had some good friends and a close relationship with my family. I was successful and satisfied, wasn't I?

Grandpa was the only person who knew better and was willing to call me on it. "It's too late for me, but it's not too late for you." He said it out of love for me, with his own sincere regret about what he didn't do in his own life. He knew what I was capable of, and that it was far greater than anything I'd done to date. Even as he was fading away, he provided me the energy and the impetus to climb the biggest mountain on earth.

But I'd be lying to you if I told you that I immediately set about changing my life when I got home. Instead, I kept doing the same old, same old. I told myself I'd start truly living out my dreams really soon, once things cleared up a bit—which, of course, meant I never did a thing.

It wasn't until a few months later, in February 1999, when my grandpa's suffering came to an end, that his words bored their way through my thick skull. I returned for his funeral in Tucson, at the same church where my grandpa and grandma said their vows to each other fifty-nine years earlier, and was overcome with emotion. Various family members and friends took turns going up to the pulpit to say a few words about Grandpa and relate their experiences and remembrances of him.

Finally, it was my turn. I had prepared a few stories that I considered worth sharing, but now they seemed somewhat trivial and inappropriate. With his recent words still singing in my ears, I poured out my heart and let everyone know how much my grandfather had affected my life, and how much he continued to affect it. It was a time for fond remembrances, but also for truth.

"I have had many male influences in my life, many men that I have admired.

They have all let me down one way or another, except one: my grandpa. He never, ever disappointed me," I said.

Then I began to cry. But to try to offset the tremendous sadness I was feeling, I also began to laugh and smile. As I continued to talk, his last words to me finally anchored themselves to my soul: "I will from now on, until the day I die, live every day as if it's my last. Every adventure I perform will be in his honor."

I reached down and grabbed a bottle of Aquavit (which means "water of life"), the Scandinavian liquor that our Norwegian family members toast with. I poured the Aquavit into a shot glass that my grandfather had used and raised it to the audience. "To you, Grandpa. Skål," I said, and I gulped the liquid down.

I believe, to this day, that those two ounces of Aquavit just might have contained my grandfather's spirit, because by the time I returned to the pew I silently vowed to strike out for the big goal that had occupied my daydreams over the previous four years: climbing Mount Everest. I was not going to let fear and doubt kill any of my dreams anymore, and I suddenly was determined to take others with me, even if I had to carry them part of the way. At the end of what I hoped would be a very long life, I wanted to gaze back and know deep within myself that I had no regrets, no missed opportunities, no dreams unfulfilled.

It's no exaggeration to say I never would have climbed Everest, established a world record on Kilimanjaro, won a marathon at the North Pole, or even had this book published, without my grandfather's inspiration.

Is there someone in your family who's inspired you in a similar way? If not, that's okay; I would like to offer myself as that person to you. Not merely as the guy who helped you lose the ten or thirty pounds, helped you stop drinking, overeating, or acting in other self-destructive ways, or motivated you to compete in a century bike race—but also as the man who encouraged you to really get in touch with yourself, discover what you want out of life, and learn the ways of getting there.

My grandfather made me see the light, and Hyperfitness can do the same for you. You can learn to live every moment in life to the fullest and treat life like the gift that it is. It's never too late. I wish I'd seen that light a lot earlier, but I am thankful to see it every day now. Whether you're a teenager or older adult, or somewhere in between, you may wish that you'd read this book a lot earlier. But don't look back and live with regret. Resolve to go forward—from wherever you are right now, from whatever shape you're in, from any unpleasant situation you're a part of—and do great things, for yourself, for your loved ones, for the community you live in, for the world.

You're on earth to do something, and something very important. Are you doing it now? If so, great—here's a program to help you do it even better. And if you're stuck in mediocrity, with mediocre goals, Hyperfitness Living will jolt you right out of it. Simply put, if you follow the program, even part of the program, your life will have no choice but to improve in every way. You will be fitter, feel better, look better, have more energy, achieve more goals, be mentally stronger, and have more faith in yourself—and that'll be only the tip of the iceberg.

It didn't hit me until the day my grandpa died—why *can't* I climb Mount Everest? It's the same question you should ask of yourself, no matter how big a goal you're going to pursue. "Why can't I _____?" It's simple: Believe that you can, then act upon those beliefs, and you will.

I began this book four years ago because I wanted others to read it and be inspired, just like the students in my fitness classes.

Reading how to reach your dream goals is one issue; actually being able to take that information presented to you and go out and do it is another. Don't be that person who reads but does not act, has the vision for the goal but does not follow through, is willing but lets himself or herself get sidetracked.

For so long, that was me: the dreamer, the reader, the observer. I'd leave it to someone else to climb the mountain, to get the message out, to do good in the world. I didn't think that I could make a difference. I was afraid of change, of losing the comforts of life, like the car and the house.

One day, a few months after returning from the highs of Everest to my consulting job, I told my wife that I couldn't do what I was doing anymore. I was making close to $100,000, but I was miserable. She, on her monster salary from teaching elementary school, smiled and said, "I support you, sweetheart, in whatever you decide to do." Since then, the ceiling on my happiness level has been raised because I started doing what I wanted with my life, and once the work started to pay off—the Everest climb, the North Pole Marathon record win, the record ascent of Mount Kilimanjaro, motivational speaking to companies, fitness consulting, this book being published—I went through the roof right over that ceiling! The sky was the limit, literally. I want you, too, to take the roof right off the glass ceiling of your dreams, and walk on the roof of the world!

Through years of work with clients ranging widely in their fitness and motivation levels—from the once active individual who hasn't been able to drop those extra fifteen pounds, to the "weekend warrior" who wants to take his or her training to a new level, to the person who's given up every previous attempt at getting into shape—I have seen, firsthand, the effects of Hyperfitness, and how they are different from those of any other program out there. I have seen how Hyperfitness goes far beyond the "cosmetic effect" of a leaner and stronger body, and boosts many other areas in my clients' lives, including family, career, education, spirituality, recreation, and social outreach.

By sharing the experiences of clients who have succeeded beyond their wildest dreams to conquer their own Inner Everests (you'll find out a lot more about these later), whether it's climbing a volcano in Mexico, running a half-marathon, participating in an adventure race, or even starting to earn a living in a manner you have yet to fathom, I will show you that it's never too late to change your life and join the ranks of those who have begun Hyperfitness.

Are you ready for a twelve-week journey of self-discovery and self-realization that will transform you, both mentally and physically? Even if you're not ready to shout an enthusiastic "yes!" yet, you will once you notice your increased energy levels and improved body shape, along with a renewed commitment to go out and truly follow your dreams. If that seems overly ambitious for a twelve-week program, have some faith in me! My years of experience as an internationally recognized fitness trainer and world-record-setting athlete have shown me that people of any fitness level can absolutely transform themselves in such a time period given the right attitude, the right physical training, and the right nutritional guidelines.

This book is not simply a fitness or exercise manual, a nutritional primer, a motivational book, or a book about how to scale a mountain; it's a guide to how you can achieve a whole new meaningful life.

I have high hopes for you, too. I'm sure you've heard the saying "Everything happens for a reason." Have you ever felt that there was a mystical, guiding force directing you in life? I have, and I've written this book to pass along that sense of being in sure hands to others. Stay with me, friend, and I will guide you every step of the way. I thank you for giving me your trust and hope, and I promise to return the favor in ways that neither of us can yet imagine.

Chapter 1

THE DREAM

Do you remember a time in your life when your body was conditioned, your mind was sharp, and you felt like you were on top of the world? That describes Hyperfitness perfectly, and it extends far beyond any other program you may have tried or read or heard about. In fact, it isn't just a series of unusual workouts, a nutritional regimen, or a method for achieving a perfect-looking body, or even the strongest and most athletic one. It is all those things, sure, but it is also a great deal more: It offers a template for approaching and overcoming all of your life's challenges.

It may sound outrageous, but you may learn more about yourself in the next twelve weeks than in your entire life to date, no matter what your age. I've seen it happen countless times with clients, because they put in the work and got the results they had been wanting to see and experience for years, such as wearing clothes that hadn't fit them in a decade, becoming more athletic than ever before, and possessing an unreal energy level that carried over to everything they did each day. What they didn't expect, though, is how Hyperfitness allowed them to achieve major turnarounds in the most important areas of their lives. They renewed their outlook on life, forged or mended relationships with loved ones, created better career prospects, reversed health problems, and even found a bigger role for themselves on this planet. In every way, it drastically improved their lives.

If you could embark upon a journey that would take your life to such unprecedented heights, you'd go, right? This book is your chance. A few years ago, you wouldn't have found me so fired up. Instead, I was plodding away on life's treadmill: getting up every day feeling trapped, going to a job I didn't like, and having no one to share the few good things in my life with.

What's in the Name "Hyperfitness"?

In case you've already met me or seen me on TV, you may suspect that Hyperfitness got its tag from my hyper self. Sorry to disappoint, but the name was coined by a writer who wrote a feature about my fitness training for the *Washington Post Magazine*. After watching a couple of my classes, she threw out the word "hyperfitness," because I had told her the term "extreme fitness" didn't conjure up the right images for the style of exercises I had developed. My classes are kinetic all the time, always doing new moves, combining all the muscles, taking almost no rest, shouting out mantras, and generally getting in a phenomenal workout—while having a great time.

I wasn't done, though, because Hyperfitness is a lot more than a particular brand of workout. As any of my students can tell you, it's a lifestyle that extends from your newly created self, with an energetic body, tireless mind, and indefatigable spirit.

Many people go through life waiting for things to happen to them, for dreams to come true, for money to fill their pockets, for someone to whisk them off their feet. Their days might begin strong, with big thoughts and great expectations, but close with little to show for themselves besides shelved and unfulfilled ideas. Does that sound extreme? The idea might seem outlandish at first—but when you take an unflinching look at yourself, you'll see many grains of truth. I certainly did. I was in a day-to-day battle with decisions and disappointments, physical highs and lows, positive and negative moods, dreams created and then lost—and I was losing.

I was wish-fishing with nothing on the line. I forgot that for good things, and especially great ones, to happen to, and for, you, you've got to put in the effort and be willing to shake things up. Until that day, I wasn't ready to alter my life.

You see, dreams give life hope, meaning, and purpose. They put the light on in the room. But then it's up to you to do something in that room to make that dream a reality. Do that workout, call that potential business partner, write that song. Living a fulfilled life is essentially dream-chasing, putting into action the hopes you have for yourself, your loved ones, or your community.

The first step, of course, is to introduce that dream into reality by rejecting the box that others may want to put you in. In life people are often given roles to play—the obedient son, the all-star pupil, or perhaps the unconditional corporate team player. And like many of the roles you see in the movies, it's *not* your role of a lifetime; instead, it's as limiting as the story line that surrounds your character.

Don't limit yourself to what you want to do. Why can't you do what you dream of doing—start a local clothing company, learn to play the guitar, run a restaurant, or compete in a triathlon? Don't underestimate yourself. People are always going to underestimate you, but you need to stop doing it to yourself. People want others to be miserable because sometimes *they're* miserable, so you must realize that their behavior has got *nothing* to do with you. If you suddenly became successful in whatever you're trying to achieve, they'd get uncomfortable, and people don't like being uncomfortable so they try to sabotage you, oftentimes innocently. "Can't you work out tomorrow instead?" "Majoring in that subject makes no sense for you." "Starting in this kind of business has just too much risk attached." "Are you sure you don't want fries with that?"

Maybe you had the misfortune to have people in your life who basically gave you messages that created limitations, or told you that you'd never amount to anything. Well, those are some serious shackles to shake off, but instead of letting such hurdles become boundaries, keep your dream alive. Who knows, maybe they'll understand you better once you achieve it.

Do Away with Doubt

So many of the great things that you do in life happen during those fleeting, unpredictable moments when you decide to cross the room to talk with someone who may be your future love, to study the subject in college that your parents don't endorse, or to start writing a book even though you know nothing about how to get it published (hint: that was me in that last example!). Push the destructive visitor of doubt out of your life. Instead, make a decision to trust your positive instincts rather than your negative ones; be impetuous, daring, and confident. When I am exercising, teaching, on an expedition, or in a business meeting, I never doubt my beliefs and what I can accomplish as a human being. I know that if doubt enters my mind, the objective I am trying to achieve may fail. You must believe in yourself 150 percent.

For example, some of you are already saying, "Am I cut out for this program?" or "It looks too hard." That's doubt getting the best of you, or more likely robbing you until you're blind and bloated. Say "Yes, I can do this!" Say "This will improve my life in every way!" And, by all means, feel free to yell it out loud. Your mind and body need that wake-up call.

Learn to Be Fit

Changing your life for good starts with learning to be at your full potential physically. I'm not condescending to you when I tell you, "Learn to be fit." To me, ceasing to learn is the same as ceasing to live. You need to keep learning and practicing how to incorporate different exercises and ways of eating into your life. It's a vigilant process, but this book will make that process a lot easier for you, as long as you're willing to soak up the information like a sponge!

Every day, I wake up ready to learn more: from my family; my clients; other people I run across; the things I read and see. Many people, though, might have shut off that process, saying, essentially, that "Life is what it is—I have my job and my kids, and I'll just wait until they graduate and then I'll do something about learning how to make my dreams more of a reality." Or: "My habits are what they are, as is my routine." So, as they age, their habits and routines push them downhill until their dreams are buried and forgotten.

In the workout arena, I guarantee you will learn to exercise in a more radically different, more exciting way than you ever have before. If you have any bad feelings about exercise, Hyperfitness will obliterate them along with your fat stores. If you're currently on some sort of regular exercise program that just isn't doing the job for you anymore, physically and/or mentally, then this is just the ticket. As health club memberships rise, so do the burnout cases. Gym owners, especially the big chains, know this well, for they will accept far more members than could possibly fit into their spaces, knowing that a sizable percentage will stop coming sooner or later.

For the people who do manage to get in their workouts much of the time, maintaining regular exercise and a healthy lifestyle is a battle or chore. They may be strengthening their muscles or cardiovascular systems, but they aren't reaching their maximum potential physically, or fueling their bodies properly and building mental fortitude. They may be doing a reasonably effective routine, but it's one without much variety and it's guaranteed to have one end result: boredom. So many people need a realistic program that not only works for them but also generates the good feeling and results they'll need to stick to it for a lifetime.

That program didn't exist until now, with this book, and that's a boast that I can back up. I've read the other books, and I've seen countless personal trainers work out their clients. And their programs either fail to inspire—since the exercise routine becomes too dull or the diet becomes too hard to follow, so you can't achieve lasting results—or the programs ask your body to undergo an ordeal that isn't really natural, like stripping carbohydrates from your diet or requiring you to plod along in your jogging shoes for miles every workout. Eventually both your body and mind rebel, and say, "Forget this!"

In this book, I will reveal to you the program I developed that eventually allowed me to meet my dream goal, which was to climb Everest. But your dream may be different from mine. At the start of the program, you will determine your own Inner Everest, or goals for the program.

At speaking engagements, I have been asked numerous times: "Where did you get this information?" "What books do you read?" "How did you come up with these theories that proved to be so successful?" It was an answer that was so easy, but it took my grandfather's death for me to realize what it was. Experiencing life! That's the answer. And I don't mean just moving through life, living day to day, living for the weekends or vacation. No, I am speaking about living each moment as if it were your last.

I'm asking you to read, think passionately, act with no regrets, and embrace the Hyperfitness program for twelve weeks. If you do this, your life will begin to reach extraordinary heights. You will meet your dream goals, and the journey to these goals along the way will truly define who you are as a person inside, which is really all we ever desire to know about ourselves.

The Three Pieces of the Puzzle

Now that I've explained that this is not just another fitness book, let's go over the three crucial components that make up Hyperfitness: Hyperstrength, Hyperfare, and Hypermind. Each element relies, and builds upon, the other, and to reach your full potential in all aspects of your life you need to make a commitment to incorporating all three into your daily existence. The Hypermind component is the lynchpin for the entire program. As you will see, possessing a Hypermind makes it possible to follow the Hyperstrength workouts and Hyperfare eating plans.

Develop Hyperstrength

If a Hypermind is the lynchpin, then **Hyperstrength** is the nuts and bolts. I will provide step-by-step instructions for strength and cardiovascular training and guide you every step of the way through the drills and exercises regardless of your current fitness level. I originally designed many of these exercises for both myself and my students, and the emphasis was on making them effective and original, as in no isolation moves and no same-old moves! Did I hear a sigh of relief?

I've taught Hyperfitness classes for twelve years now and have practiced martial arts for eighteen years. I've dealt with hundreds of students and know that you are no different from them. You can handle this program, so don't doubt yourself. I want you to reach your potential, and Hyperstrength will help you get there physically. I sometimes hear that my program pushes too hard or even that I'm crazy. That makes me laugh. These comments always come from people who have never tried the program—as we know, it's much easier to criticize than to exercise!

Almost all fitness programs suffer from three big problems for the exerciser: 1) whether the architect was aware of it or not, they're based upon bodybuilding principles; 2) they give you the same exercises again and again until you're bored silly; and 3) they are not well-rounded in their approach to get you in shape. In other words, they're probably not designed with you and your goals in mind—far from it—and you're likely to quit the program at some point over frustration at the lack of progress or simple boredom.

Bodybuilding principles include isolating the muscle groups, using split routines in which you work only part of the body on each training day, relying on exercise machines (the majority of which, again, isolate your muscles), taking long rests between sets, and spending most of the training time lifting weights. A lot of women, for instance, are unwittingly put on bodybuilding-like programs by personal trainers without knowing it. But bodybuilding is designed for one thing and one thing only: to make your muscles bigger. If that's your number-one workout goal—muscle size, and not strength, speed, function, or athleticism—then by all means use a bodybuilding-type plan. Most of us, however, want to look athletic, lean, strong, and fit rather than bulging, juiced, or vascular. More important than the look, we want to *be* athletic, *be* able to run after our kid in the backyard, *be* equipped to easily cycle up a huge hill or compete in any fitness event.

Other fitness programs almost always rely on the same exercises, and you're naturally going to be less and less inspired to do four sets of lunges after a while, no matter how good they are for you. Last, targeting all of your muscle fibers, building muscle balance, working your core, incorporating flexibility, developing speed, and improving cardiovascular performance are *all* important elements of a workout program. Most routines only hit one or two of these areas.

Hyperstrength is a program for you if you want to reach your maximum potential and be athletic, lean, and strong. Every two weeks I'll show you new exercises that will challenge your body and help you reap all the benefits of exercise.

And that's exactly the point, as I want you to push muscles in new ways and along the way begin to realize something new about yourself. You will find that your workouts can even approach a spiritual experience, helping to instill a greater belief in yourself.

The Hyperstrength program includes foundation building, muscle balance and agility, core strengthening, plyometrics (explosive movement training), heart-rate zone training and cardiovascular conditioning, real-life integrated strength concepts, sport-specific drills, and flexibility. Even better, you're not going to be focusing on one training element at a time, like the typical program in which you strengthen a part of the body for a while, then another part, then the abs, then some cardio, and so on. You couldn't pay me to do that type of program, nor will I ask it of you. Instead, the Hyperstrength program trains all the muscles in your body at once! So, yes, it will be tough, especially in the beginning, but your gains in strength, fat loss, agility, speed, and overall athleticism will astound you, especially because they will occur rapidly. Hyperstrength is about creating a body ready for real-world adventures.

Exercises are divided into warm-ups, which include basic exercises like squats with knee lifts, jumping jacks, and standing alternating toe touches; phase exercises, like speed-skating drills, squatting canoe rows using a body bar, and step/box variations; and my pioneering Inner Everest (IE) drills. IE drills are uniquely designed exercise sequences consisting of a series of varying high-intensity moves. These innovative integrated challenges will stretch you both physically and mentally, and keep you absorbed in the program. In other words, I will give you some staple exercises like jumping rope that you will master, and I will also throw in some completely new exercises or drills that will bring up your fitness level. I've found that the combination of a few familiar moves with some unfamiliar ones is not only how you improve, but also how you stay interested.

At the heart of Hyperstrength is my belief in rigorous training, so I'm asking you to devote ½ hour to 1½ hours per day, five or six days per week, depending on your fitness level. And I'll vary your workout routine every two weeks to further amp up your body's rate of conditioning and prevent any staleness before it starts.

While the Hyperstrength program will work for any type of individual regardless of age or current fitness level, I've made it easier to begin by providing three levels: Trekkers, Climbers, and Sherpas.

Which Fitness Level Currently Describes You?

Each of you currently exists at a certain level of strength and endurance, so it only makes sense to choose the level that best suits you now. Be careful not to overshoot in the beginning and choose too high a level, because it could cause excessive muscle soreness, burnout, and potential injury. I recommend that if anything you underestimate your current fitness shape, so staying on the program remains realistic. If you stick with the program, you will make it to the Sherpa level. The formula is very simple: effort directly determines the result, meaning, if you put in the time and effort, you will make dramatic progress.

Because Hyperstrength is not your normal fitness program, though, you might even choose to remain at the Trekker or Climber levels, or occasionally to return to those levels when you have less time that week or need more recovery time. All levels have their purpose and contain excellent, unique exercises and drills. For example, simply by upping the poundage to be lifted, adding sets, or lowering rest times, a Sherpa can get a great workout from the Trekker program.

Trekkers: These are folks who probably were active when they were younger but have pushed exercise and nutrition to the periphery of their lives. They have not made fitness a priority for quite some time and perhaps think it is too late or too difficult to get back into the kind of shape they were once in. Or they're individuals who have never exercised aside from recreational walking and those long-ago P.E. classes. Well, I will reintroduce Trekkers to the rewards of a fit body and mind by showing them exactly what they can accomplish in only twelve weeks of physical and mental training.

Climbers: Climbers are people who have made a partial commitment to a healthier lifestyle by staying active and watching their weight, but have not been pleased with their results. They exercise somewhat sporadically, consider staying fit a chore, and lack the proper resolve to stick with it. What they need, and what Hyperfitness offers them, is a rigorous and rewarding fitness program with creative incentives to keep them motivated.

Sherpas: Sherpas are individuals who want to become the finest conditioned athletes around. They exercise on a consistent basis every week, desire to work toward higher levels of fitness, and are looking for the right guide to help them reach their potential. They feel comfortable around all types of fitness equipment and are able to exercise at an endurance pace several days a week. They also watch what they eat and tend to be competitive within themselves and in other areas of life. For everything they are doing right, however, Sherpas understand that they cannot realize their potential and reach their goals—such as ocean marathons, the Ironman, and climbing Everest—without the guidance of a professional trainer.

Starting with Chapter Three, you will find a two-week workout for each level at the end of each chapter. Although you probably are anxious to start the physical program, I highly recommend that you read the first three chapters before beginning the Hyperstrength portion.

Again, in the interest of making this program accessible to all, many of the exercises/drills can be done without a gym membership or access to equipment. If you mostly work out at home, you can select drills that use boxed platforms or minimal equipment, such as a jump rope, dumbbells, or a medicine ball. If you go to a gym or have bought additional home equipment (such as a pull-up bar and a Swiss ball), you may choose drills that take advantage of the full range of equipment available.

Consume Hyperfare

My recommendations for eating—called **Hyperfare**—are an essential piece of your new evolution. The last thing you need to hear is that you should give up carbohydrates and start consuming massive amounts (and spending just as much) of some supplement with my name on it. Instead, I encourage you to return to a better way of eating, starting with purchasing foods that require you to use a kitchen, preferably yours.

The top four reasons Americans have gotten so obese these days are 1) packaged foods, many of which are completely unhealthy; 2) an apparent cooking allergy, replaced by the "I'll pick up something on the way home, honey" syndrome; 3) out-of-control portion sizes, which often go undetected because of the mammoth plates and vessels that our food and drink are doled out in, along with the mammoth restaurant meals averaging about 1,500 calories; and 4) snacking on foods loaded with calories but containing zero nutrition—like chips, candies, doughnuts, and cookies—and that usually make you want to do one thing: eat more. All four reasons add up to hundreds of more calories per day and pounds of fat per year, and it explains why even those who exercise frequently are stuck in permanent physical plateaus.

A lot of our eating habits come from a quick-fix mentality. We can't help ourselves from buying the prepackaged, processed food that keeps us from cooking and actually sitting down and enjoying a meal with our loved ones. Instead, we eat while we are driving, snack while we watch TV or work at our desks, and grab lunch on the go, hardly noticing what we slam into our mouths. Yet our bodies were not designed to digest processed imitation foods, and we'll never see optimal results from a fitness program if we don't fuel our bodies with healthy, whole foods.

With that in mind, I have created a nutritional program called Hyperfare, which addresses our body's needs as well as taste buds—and it works with the Hypermind and Hyperstrength regimens to maximize results. I will explain the value of good proteins, like wild salmon and organic chicken breast; "clean" carbohydrates, like organic whole-grain cereals and multigrain bread; organic vegetables, like mustard greens and tomatoes, and the importance of eating vegetables in season; and healthy fats, which can be found in olive oil, flaxseed oil, all-natural peanut butter, and avocados. I will explain why organic, seasonal, locally produced food is the best way to go for your body as well as the planet. I will discuss the revival of the three-main-meals (rather than the five or six that so many other books trumpet but end up simply causing their readers confusion and overeating) tradition, including the old idea that breakfast should be your biggest meal of the day.

I will also talk about the difficult issue of snacking, and how you don't need to abstain from eating between meals altogether, but need to make intelligent choices. I'll recommend snack foods that help diminish hunger pains until the next meal, and give you my favorite recipes. By following my Hyperfare guidelines, you will look better, feel better, and optimize your Hyperfitness results.

Get a Hypermind

The final piece of the puzzle is **Hypermind,** and it's what locks everything into place. The Hypermind program is adapted from my nearly two decades of martial arts training. Mastery of these principles will allow you to not only control your fears but also to use them in a positive fashion to continue moving toward your goals. You will learn to increase your energy in order to become more powerful internally, become calm and energetic rather than stressed out, adapt to any trying circumstances that you are faced with, reduce your large goals down to smaller and more manageable tasks, persist through challenges once dismissed as being unfeasible, and continue to expand mentally for the rest of your life.

Maybe you're thinking, "Whoa, those are a lot of promises." Well, if you promise to follow this program, all that will happen, and more. Physically you can undergo wonderful changes with the aid of Hyperstrength and Hyperfare alone, but a Hypermind helps you whenever your energy is flagging and your drive is wanting. Beyond the physical goals, including getting to the literal and metaphorical places in your life where you really want to be, a Hypermind brings all of them within range.

How did you feel when you woke up this morning? Were you excited for the day to begin, or did you want to crawl under the blankets and sleep the day away? Do you greet each circumstance with energy and thoughtfulness, or do you simply go through the motions until you arrive back in front of the TV or join your friends at the bar? It's amazingly easy to forget the miracle of life and let the minutes slip away with little to show for ourselves as the years pile up. Grim, right? You don't want that to be your life!

Listen, I'm not up on the mountaintop preaching down to you. I created this program because I needed it just as much as or more than you do, so I'm preaching to myself as well. Exercise saved me, eating healthy foods made me feel better, and learning to think positively and productively finally gave me a future worth fighting for. At the same time, I gradually developed some spiritual strength that would get me through the inevitable low points, because developing yourself spiritually truly gives you a complete Hypermind.

It's all linked—exercise, love, nutrition, work, spirit, fulfillment—and we forget that. We read a magazine article about how to lose five pounds through diet, watch a guru tell us how to heal our relationships, buy a DVD that will produce six-pack abs, and it mirrors the disconnected life that so many of us live. There is nothing wrong with any of those activities, but they tend to overcomplicate a life that may already be awash in chaos.

With Hyperfitness, I link it all together for you. I want to make life better for you in every way, and I also want to make it easier. A lifestyle change has a great chance of succeeding only when it begins with mental conditioning, which is why the Hypermind is the crucial first step in this program. Through visualization exercises, inspirational mantras, and centering meditations, you will gain a new mental fortitude that will empower you to identify your dreams and achieve them. These psychological techniques, tested both by myself and hundreds of my clients, are sure to keep you focused on conquering your Inner Everests throughout the duration of the program, and far beyond.

The Journey Begins . . .

I'm asking you to join me on a journey to truly find yourself and to revive the vision, principle, and faith of making your dreams become reality. The first plan of action is the **self-discovery journey.**

This exercise involves finding a quiet, peaceful place, ideally outdoors on a sunny day. You might hike to the summit of a small mountain that offers unobstructed views, take a walk on a beach at sunset, find a lake or river that is off the beaten path, or simply choose an isolated spot in a park. This location should be one that you've never been to before so the experience is completely new to your senses, and you should go alone. Once you reach your destination, sit down and take in a few deep breaths. Close your eyes and listen to the sounds that you hear. After a few minutes, open your eyes and look carefully at the nature around you. Place your hands in the sand, roll your fingers over a stone, feel the breeze against your face. I want you to see, smell, hear, and feel everything around you—everything but your life back at home and at work. For fifteen minutes, breathe deeply and softly; try to remain as peaceful as possible while you are doing this. Literally let time stand still in your mind and let only the surroundings in.

Next, think about your dreams and the goals you want to achieve in life. It doesn't matter how insane, sane, or farfetched they are. These dreams and goals are yours and yours alone, so don't be influenced by how others may perceive or judge them. And I'm not talking about the "lose ten pounds" goal, which is legitimate, of course, but is a small goal compared to what I'm talking about. For example, many people lose their goal weight but then get stuck, wondering what to accomplish next. Without larger goals and, thus, motivation, they inevitably start slacking off. It's essential that *you* dig deeper.

How about being healthy for a lifetime? Making a big contribution to society? Raising healthy and happy children? Maybe doing a full Ironman triathlon, building your own house, beginning your own company, quitting smoking, sailing around the world, writing a book, recovering from heart surgery (like my client Daniel D.; see page 19), developing a more intimate marriage, becoming a complete athlete, climbing Everest!

You, and you alone, are the sole benefactor of your fate. Life is how *you* look at it, and how you treat it.

Try to think beyond yourself when you're creating your dream goals. Think

Expand Your Horizons by Expanding Your Goals

It's easy to get fixated on only one goal, and many people live day after day without any real goal at all. To help you come up with more goals, write down at least one for each of the following: a charitable goal, a personal goal, a creative goal, a spiritual goal, a physical goal, and a family goal.

It's a way of finding out who exactly you are by getting you away from the role you play in your daily life. It boils down to what is truly important to you and might even cause you to notice that you didn't have goals in many of these categories.

of your loved ones and the less fortunate, and you may begin to see how much you can do for both them and yourself. Reflect on goals that will involve you on a journey that you've never taken before. The journey is when you learn things about yourself, and when you grow, struggle, and succeed.

For me, Everest became a journey I had to take in order to become the kind of man I wanted to be, one who could truly help others. During my expeditions, I've seen so much suffering in the world and the daunting challenges that everyday living poses for many people. Now I could never be content with just reaching goals and breaking records—my frame of reference has expanded by many orders of magnitude. So aim high and wide. Affect many besides yourself and you will be truly fulfilled.

Once you come up with a dozen or so dream goals, write them down in your personal **Hyperfitness journal.** First, see them in your mind, then whisper them softly to yourself, and then read each dream goal out loud a few times. Each time you repeat your dream goal, voice it a little louder until finally you are yelling each one of them as loud as you possibly can. So loud the heavens can hear you. (Now do you understand why I suggested finding a very private spot in nature?)

From the dream goals you have written down, choose one big goal that you want to achieve above all others and that you think you can achieve if you harness all your energy and power for an extended period of time. It should also define who you are and/or who you want to be. Once you have chosen a goal, this one will be your big **Inner Everest** to achieve. Congratulations on your choice. Now let's start working together to achieve it!

In the later, more challenging, phases of the Hyperfitness program, the very existence of this long-term goal will keep you focused and motivated. It will maximize your chances of long-term success and of transforming that dream into action.

Short-term Goals Will Lead the Way

Are you ready to embark on your Inner Everest expedition? I want you to leave symbolically the comfort of your old life, your routines, and come with me to Nepal, where together we will climb the highest peak in the world, Mount Everest.

Almost all Everest climbs commence in Kathmandu, at 4,344-feet elevation at the foothills of the Himalayas. It's the largest city in Nepal, a small country tucked between China and India. By the time you reach Kathmandu, your body already begins to be deprived of oxygen and tries to compensate by a process known as altitude acclimatization. At sea level, your body functions at its best because your red blood cells get abundant oxygen, close to 100 percent; as you make your way up the mountain, additional red blood cells are created, your heart beats faster, and you start to breath more frequently and deeply.

However, as is true of the Hyperfitness journey, acclimatization takes time and you're advised to climb no more than 2,000 feet on any given day. Sometimes, for acclimatization and training purposes, you may do a trekking hike and spend the night in the same spot from which you started. At 17,600 feet, or the height of base camp, your natural oxygen supply has been cut in half, so you need to spend at least two weeks to allow your body to adapt. Overall, it takes about a month to acclimatize fully in order to make a summit attempt, and the entire Everest journey usually takes two and a half months, which can be a long time to be away from your loved ones. Similarly, each Hyperstrength phase lasts two weeks, you'll find a groove in about a month, and the entire program will be twelve weeks.

I have lived my entire life at sea level, which makes climbing the big mountains that much more difficult. You, too, may have figuratively lived at sea level in regard to your exercise adventures, so you're about to face a similar challenge. But the greater the distance you must travel, the sweeter the arrival.

The long-term, Inner Everest goal is the mountaintop that you can see in the distance, but you also need **short-term goals** to keep you motivated for the next twelve weeks and beyond. You will also want to select short-term goals that are realistic to achieve by the thirteenth week, as twelve weeks is not enough training time for a triathlon or growing time for an organic farm, for instance. In fact, the long-term IE goal may take you two, four, or several more years precisely because it is so large, so you have to develop your own stepping stones along the way that are consistent with that big goal. (It took me five years to get to Everest once I put it on my map.) So maybe do a spring warm-up for the triathlon. Or perhaps the short-term goal that will get you closer to your Inner Everest is getting a promotion, taking the next step in your relationship, or beginning to learn rock-climbing skills.

You should have certain **physical short-term** goals along the way, in terms of performance (from knocking a minute off your mile time to your ability to put on previously too-tight clothing) and appearance (from a thinner waistline by burning off that jiggled fat deposit, to getting that lean, strong silhouette that you've always craved). Look, I'm not going to judge you on any of your goals. I want you to be the best possible person that you can be and reach your maximum potential on this earth.

Make Your Dreams a Reality

Every day, ask yourself this question: "Am I using a portion of this day to make my dream become reality?" That question helps guide me and gets me thinking about what I am doing and how I am spending my time. Am I approaching anything? Getting anywhere? Am I working for that goal or did I waste that time? Did I just laze out and eat junk? Was it worth it? Couldn't I have put in a great day and finished it with a filling healthy meal and great conversation?

Ask yourself questions, and then act on the answers to those questions. Don't be complacent. I am constantly fed the line "Wow, I wish I were in your kind of shape." My answer is always, "You can be!" No one shook magic exercise dust over my head. I am just like anyone else. I just made the decision for action instead of wishful thinking. It is always your choice. You can read this book or not, you can be active or lazy, and you can chase that dream or give up. You know what you need to do.

Remember, the most important facet of your dream goal is the journey and not the actual goal being attained. That's when you learn and change as a person. If you stay centered, committed, and open to each step and experience, you will grow more than you ever thought possible.

Beyond the symbolism, there's another reason for making this program twelve weeks: a month is simply too easy, and so many give up after that. In three months, you will see incredible results. If you can commit to Hyperfitness that long, you will be able to reach your goals and accomplish anything you set your mind to. It will get the program into your blood—and if I can get you committed for three months, you can be dedicated for life.

Hyperfitness is not about luck—it's about your dreams, your desire, and your ability to commit and work hard with a smile on your face. Don't be subpar, like I was for too long. Reach your potential and bring others with you.

Daniel D., Fifty-seven, Engineer

Daniel began Hyperfitness four months after undergoing quadruple bypass surgery.

"Although I had no symptoms, based on my family history of heart disease, my primary physician ordered a stress test as part of a physical in July 2002. The test results were abnormal, which subsequently led to immediate additional tests scheduled as soon as feasible. The nuclear stress test and angiogram that followed resulted in a diagnosis of coronary artery disease and revealed four coronary arteries more than 90 percent blocked. I underwent quad bypass surgery on September 3, 2002, at the age of fifty-three.

"I returned to work approximately eight weeks after surgery, although full recovery and a return to near normal took quite a bit longer. There were both physical and mental challenges to all that went on, and while I consider myself very lucky (to be alive, to be with my family, to have had a good family doctor, to be healthy), it is an ordeal that I urge all to avoid. Unlike many, I wanted to exercise post-surgery during cardiac rehabilitation, which I did on my own. Four months post-surgery, I could not do a single sit-up because of latent incision pain and muscle atrophy.

"My real progress since the surgery has come since January 2005, when I started training under the direction of Sean Burch's Hyperfitness program. For me, the results have been extraordinary. Even with the beta blocker I take every day (which suppresses the fight or flight response, makes you tire more quickly, and reduces your heart rate by 10–20 bpm), in training with Sean I've raised my AT [anaerobic threshold] by some 20–25 bpm over what it was when I started the class, my overall cardiac fitness has increased dramatically to the point where I do things now that four to five months ago there would have been no way (warming up on the treadmill at a pace more than 2 mph faster than I could do when I started and leaping multiple times onto steps with 10 risers, in but one of the most recent examples). I enjoy a level of fitness and well-being that I have not experienced since I was a teenager. And it is not only the physical—my mind and spirit are also much better for it. Having aced the nuclear stress test last month and having my cardiologist tell me to keep doing what I am doing are just more encouragement to keep pushing forward."

Chapter 2

THE COMMITMENT

BEFORE MY EVEREST CLIMB, I TRAV-
eled from Kathmandu—the capital of Nepal—to Lukla, a two-week trek away
from the base of Everest. Upon leaving Kathmandu, I was essentially leaving behind the comforts of modern civilization, like hotel beds and showers. There was
no turning back. Sure, I was nervous, just as you may be as you head into the
Hyperfitness program.

Right out of the gate, I was tested with a harrowing plane ride into Lukla.
We landed on a cliff, literally. The pilot told us that the runway was banked up-
hill to slow the plane down more quickly because the runway is so short—this
was supposed to make us feel better.

Our tiny plane finally did slam into the runway and did a few small bounces
before coming to a stop. After I caught my breath, I got the sense that I was
someplace special.

I hope that you are beginning to feel the same way about this book. In many
ways, you are now in a position similar to what I was in then. Now is the time
to gather your equipment and prepare your mind for a journey that you've never
taken before, and you must allow yourself to trust that you will accomplish

Find a Mentor for That Dream

One early morning after a workout, an idea came to me: See if the company I worked for would give me the time off needed in order to pursue my Everest quest. I didn't wait for second thoughts, and instead marched right into my boss's office and laid out the idea. To my surprise, she agreed, and said she would do everything she could to make it a reality. Being the cool boss she was (sometimes you need a little luck, too), she lived up to her word and essentially became my mentor. She believed in me and my dreams, and this allowed me to pursue my Everest goal.

No matter what your dreams are, you probably can do with a little outside help. While many of us are too proud, shy, or lazy to ask for such help, it can make or break your chance of achieving your goals. And you may be surprised by how many good, influential people are more than willing to assist you in your pursuit.

great things as long as you stay committed. You must be ready to sweat, to crawl over obstacles, and to be unfailingly honest with yourself. Most of all, I want you to cling to your dreams and trust in yourself. Believe, with all your being, that you are capable of fulfilling your dreams.

One Flag to the Summit

After your self-discovery journey in Chapter One, you will have identified your Inner Everest goal. It's the giant one, the one that constantly makes you smile and causes you to imagine yourself fulfilled. It will help you define your purpose for living on this earth. When you identify habits of the deeply engrained thoughts or behavior you've had that have stopped you from reaching for the summit in the past—and commit to eradicating them—then your mental training begins to reach the next level.

From this point forward, until you reach the summit of your Inner Everest, every day picture achieving this goal exactly as you have envisioned it. Make it as clear as anything you have previously imagined in your life. Think of it habitually—before you go to bed at night, as soon as you wake up in the morning, and several times throughout your day. Rather than letting this dream torment you because you're not there yet, make it work for you by providing you with energy, enthusiasm, and possibility. And even if it's contrary to your nature, vocalize your dreams or goals every day, such as during your workouts and in the shower, wherever and whenever you can!

Everest was with me every day in some shape or form after I decided to commit to it—whether I was getting ready to teach my fitness classes, hiking outdoors, reading a book, or eating a meal. I was absolutely hooked on high-altitude mountaineering and now believed, fully, that I was meant to be a part of it.

You don't simply sail out and try to meet your big goals right off the bat, without first taking all necessary steps of preparation and study. Just as you wouldn't attempt to scale Everest without first climbing a small hill—then ever larger ones, with increasing degrees of difficulty and complexity—and without finding out as much as you can about how others who succeeded went about it, first, you shouldn't try running a full, 26-mile marathon without any training or experience whatsoever.

People are, generally, afraid to find out what they're made of. Granted, we all have limits, but very few of us actually ever really test them. But testing yourself mentally and physically is tremendously rewarding—why not try it? Don't be afraid to fail, and instead go for whatever goal you have. If you've never participated, say, in a half-triathlon before, you will be shocked at the tremendous boost that finishing such a race will give you.

There are too many things in life that can drag us down, but physical activity is a one-way trip in the positive direction. The Hyperfitness workouts will not only make your body healthier and stronger, they will have the same effect on your mind and even your soul. They will squash any tendency you may have to be skeptical of your abilities to reach your goals, and embolden you to see them to their final conclusion. Revel in the sweat, the toil, the physical sense of lightness that come from shucking off the weight of your everyday obligations. After those workouts, return to situations that may be causing you stress, with a clear intent on improving them, for your Hyperstrength sessions are not isolated and disconnected from the rest of your day—they are your springboard to help you embrace your life more fully.

Not too long ago my life read like a poorly conceived book, a series of mean-ingless events filling the pages. I wasn't making a significant contribution to the world or to myself, and I couldn't figure out how to get out of my rut. After I committed to climbing Everest, however, my life began to change dramatically. Each of my frequent mountaineering expeditions in preparation for the climb not only got me one step closer to my long-term goal but also became a build-ing block in the foundation of a healthier new lifestyle—and of a satisfying, ex-citing, new life.

Committing to this program can send you along the same trajectory. Follow your path to seek your Inner Everest with love for yourself and others, and you will get though any rough patches along the way. Not to be overly corny, but there is no greater force in the universe than love. And so much more can be ac-complished when you apply that force to your everyday life.

Taking Stock

At the end of Chapter One, I mentioned that short-term goals are essential in order to keep you on track for your long-term Inner Everest. Your big goal, for instance, may be a 100-mile bike race, so as a short-term goal, you might first compete in a half-century bike race. Or your physical goal could be to lose forty pounds or replace soft, fleshly limbs with lean, muscular ones, so a natural short-term goal would be to first lose ten pounds and start training to work all of your muscle fibers (in this program, you will!). Your Inner Everest goal may be to cre-ate a nonprofit agency, so as a short-term goal, you should first go about gath-ering information about public and private fundraising.

Ideally at the end of this twelve-week program, these short-term goals will be achieved, or at least bring you pretty close to getting there. Big dreamers (which I want you to be) have goals that are significant and often take some time, perhaps even many years, to achieve, so you must have a map with successful stopping points along the way. They lend a fundamental sense of accomplish-ment and keep your blood coursing through your veins; they also whet your ap-petite for making them happen.

Therefore, if you didn't do it at the end of Chapter One, jot down a short-term goal for your Inner Everest dream. Place this goal within the next three to six months, and hopefully just after the twelfth week of this program.

I had to embark on several climbs before tackling Everest to boost not just my chances of success but also of survival. (Hey, 10 percent of Everest climbers don't come back to tell their stories.) With each new expedition, I could feel myself changing, all in a good way. I began to take the lead in my own life, gained a greater appreciation for the people I cared about, and derived a deeper satisfaction from helping others and the earth.

I eventually made it to Everest because I first did Alaska, where my back-country first ascents expedition was the exact short-term goal that I needed to accomplish before I could even conceive of climbing the big one, Everest. Alone in the Alaskan wilderness, with absolutely no one to rescue me and my climbing partner if an accident or bear incident occurred—both did—we were forced to rely on our skills and strength of mind.

What Will Hyperfitness Do for You?

Hyperfitness will take you out of your comfort zone, which might even give you some preprogram jitters. That's completely natural, of course. I certainly had them before I set off for Everest, where I knew I'd face harsher weather conditions and greater body fatigue than I could even imagine. That won't happen to you here, so don't worry! But I have a hunch that you will work harder in this program than any other you've ever tried, because it's more than a body-changing program—it's life-changing.

Before you get ready to start working out, I want you to check out your current level of determination and your strengths and weaknesses. To get to your end point, it's crucial that you understand where your starting point is. Please answer these questions honestly, for you will only make it harder on yourself if you start fibbing.

Evaluating yourself will help shed light on your vulnerabilities, which you need to monitor, as well as your strengths, which you will learn to rely on.

Do you have what it takes to stay with a five-day-a-week exercise program? Can you change your eating style and limit the off-the-wagon episodes? Are you the type who will refuse to be defeated, no matter what heartbreaks befall you? Do you possess a strong spirit and creative mind but feel that you have yet to show the world what you can do?

What can you live without? Do you have to eat out at restaurants frequently, or are you willing to cook your own food most of the time? Will you be able to get a workout in before your workday starts, or can you come up with another time slot that will reliably work for you on most days?

What dreams can you live without? What are you most passionate about? At your life's end, what would you truly regret not having done?

Your Game Plan

Now you've got your goals, big and small. You know what you want, so it's time to begin plotting the way to getting there. The first pitfall that so many fall into is having no real game plan. They may have legitimate goals, but their thought process and subsequent action stops there. It's like New Year's resolutions—most people never follow through on them and within weeks, or even days, are back to their habits.

Your game plan essentially represents your path to your short-term and long-term goals. Without it you'd get lost and never wind back to those great dreams of yours. Fortunately, these goals directly involve following this program carefully, so a substantial part of your game plan is already mapped out for you. Your first job is to read this book, to follow the Hyperstrength workouts and Hyperfare eating plans, and to develop a Hypermind along the way.

Hyperfitness is preparation. Try to accept this concept with alacrity rather than reluctance. For example, don't put yourself in situations where an old habit can rear its ugly head, such as going out the door on an empty stomach (which usually sets you up to overeat at some point later) or staying up really late (which will make it extremely difficult to get in your morning workout). While other people may attempt to sabotage you, oftentimes not even consciously, by offering you food that isn't health-supportive, or encouraging you to bag the work-out, the most common saboteur is you yourself.

Don't be caught off guard. Such offers are inevitable—it isn't a question of whether they'll happen, and not even of when. You just need to be prepared and know what you will do when they come up.

So, one foot in front of the other. Every day wake up with a plan, have a plan for the week, and know what your month is going to look like. Daily and weekly events—like work, exercise, family time, food, entertainment, and errands—should be orchestrated by you, rather than having the expectation that they will just fall into place. For example, if you wake up without any real plan, you will usually miss your workout, get less work done, and even eat more poorly. So put the workout in the planner, figure out what you're going to do at work that day, and anticipate where and what you will eat that day.

No individual, or coach for that matter, can keep an entire game plan simply in his or her head, so make sure that you begin writing down your own **daily list.** If this seems unnatural or a little too obsessive, do it anyway. Trust me, you'll begin to love the practice of jotting down what you plan to do the next day on a clean pad of paper. Rather than going to bed worrying about what you *didn't* get done that day, you can revel in the satisfaction of having crossed every item off that to-do list, and note the steps you took toward your goals today. Incorporate your exercise and nutrition program goals into these daily lists, and mark down your daily progress and actions. Ideally this will all be part of your Hyperfitness journal, in which you will be able to see your progress on a daily, weekly, and monthly basis—and realize how far you've come.

Keep Positive with the Support of Others

Just as important, don't go solo with all of your goals. While it's important to be self-reliant, there are many times when a "climbing partner" or simply a friend or family member can give you the boost you need. It's crucial to cultivate relationships with people who have faith in us, and we in them; in other

Growing and Gaining Confidence in the Alaskan Backcountry

Before our Alaskan journey began, our bush pilot dropped me and my climbing partner, Chad, off in a remote area of the Wrangell–St. Elias Range. After we had gotten our gear off the single-engine Cessna 180, our pilot reached into his pocket and asked us to get in close together for a photo.

"Thanks, this will be a nice memento for after the expedition," I said.

"Oh, I didn't do this for you. If you two die up there, I want to make sure they have a picture for your family and to help claim the bodies," he said nonchalantly. Our pilot's remark sent a chill through my spine, while also instantly making our goal that much more serious. But he wasn't finished.

"You need to be here between 2 and 4 p.m., eighteen days from now. If weather is not a factor, I'll be here at 2 p.m. and wait for two hours. If you are not here and do not show up, I will assume you are both dead, and we'll get a search party going to look for you," he continued. With that, we watched him jump back into his plane and he soon took off over the trees. We stared at the now-empty sky for a few moments as I gulped down the frog in my throat.

This was serious backcountry. There were no roads, no lodges, and not even radio contact (unless a plane flew directly overhead). For two days, we crossed streams and bushwhacked our way through thicket until we reached base camp at the north face of Mount Natazhat (13,435 feet). Because of the unpredictable weather, our backpacks had supplies for every kind of weather plus all the food we needed for more than two weeks, which added up to over 100 pounds to lug around.

It was cool but freaky. One day we'd be walking in humid, suffocating air while slicing our way through chest-high thicket; the next day, we'd be walking on top of a glacier. We took full-strength bug repellent with us, but the mosquitoes and huge horseflies

words, to participate in a sharing, strong community where group goals as well as individual goals are reached. Joining a running club or a sports league, becoming an intern or taking classes, joining a neighborhood association or organizing community events puts you in good company with folks who probably have similar dreams. It's amazing what can result from that.

Not to go all Bob Marley on you, but the idea of "positive vibrations" is far more than a quaint notion. Negativity is an absolute killer, whether it's part of a family gathering, in a team setting, or on the job. I once led a group of great guys on an expedition to Mount Kilimanjaro; they were determined to have a good time, climb hard, and learn more about life. Unfortunately, this group included one negative guy who threatened to make the whole trip miserable. One day, after yet another negative outburst—complete with whiny complaints like laughed at us; I got absolutely bitten to shreds and my hands swelled up. For five straight days, we were stuck in our tent as the sky shook with thunder and poured rain, and then it snowed. Another day we stumbled across a fresh dead animal carcass that had been mauled by an unknown predator, most likely a bear.

One morning, just outside of our tent, we saw two bear cubs playing. While they were cute, it also meant that Mamma Bear was nearby. Sure enough, the next day she showed up just as we were about to leave camp for a reconnaissance trek of a mountain. She rose up on her hind legs until she was practically standing upright; sniffing the air, she stopped moving when she noticed us. Let me tell you, there's nothing like the feeling of being eyed by a creature that could easily kill you standing, literally, only fifty feet away.

Her interest piqued, she started to get closer, and I got increasingly nervous. "Chad, what do we do if she charges us?" I asked.

Chad raised his ice ax high in the air, calmly stated, "It's either us or her," and smiled from ear to ear.

This was one event I had not prepared for, so I sat there frozen until Chad started to speak calmly to her as we slowly backed away. Fortunately, she apparently thought we weren't worth a meal, so she headed back toward her cubs.

By the time the pilot came back to pick us up, I'd dropped fifteen pounds and looked like hell. But guess what? I was happy as can be. When we walked into the nearest town from the tiny airport where our pilot dropped us off for some pizza and microbrewed beer, I felt as if I had survived a physical and spiritual journey like no other. I learned how much I could take, which was an important thing for me to find out, as I knew Everest would be even harder. We also reached the summits of three peaks that had never been ascended before, which was totally thrilling.

"Why are we doing this?" and "When are we going to get there?"—I calmly said to him, "What's up with you, man? You have been negative since day one. It's time to get real—look around and enjoy this." Amazingly, he listened and turned his energy around, and he even reached the summit.

I had several people close to me telling me that I was "crazy" and "too old" to climb Everest, and even one who said "You're not going to be able to do it, Sean." I turned such negativity into fuel, which is what many great athletes excel at. Do you think Lance Armstrong or Michael Jordan let the negativity get to them? On the contrary, they fed off that stuff to make them even greater. If you can't get negative people in your life to become more positive, then keep your distance. If that's not possible, then do your best to not take any of that junk on board.

Don't be shy about sharing your dreams with your "positive" pals. In particular, tell them about your Inner Everest quest as well as your short-term goals. Encourage them to join you on a similar Hyperfitness journey, perhaps by showing them this book or simply telling them about the strides that you're making. I've found that rather than being a detriment, going public with your goals actually helps your chances of succeeding because it enforces your commitment to these goals. Don't ever forget the expression "You're only as good as your word." All of us want to be true to our word and keep our promises, so make sure that you also mention your short-term goals rather than promising a major accomplishment within an unrealistic time frame. Don't be one of the many who love to talk about their upcoming accomplishments, commitments, and promises, but cannot deliver. Do not be this person! And if you ever resemble such a person, work actively to create more realistic goals with realistic timelines.

If your current goal is "I'm going to lose thirty pounds and run a 10K." Great! Now get people around you who will say "You can do it!" Get people that you admire for their own accomplishments and drive. Before I set out for Everest, students and clients who shared similar interests and levels of dedication constantly spurred me on. In addition, find heroes who you relate to and attack life every day. Maybe it's a particular athlete or writer or musician who matches their great work with great words and subsequent action.

Getting to the Bottom of Who You Are

It may sound intense, but what I really want you to think about is **what you want out of life before you die.** Stay with me here: The purpose behind this exercise is to cement your goals over your soul and eliminate any wavering about committing to the program. For some, no matter how many great things are promised them if they accomplish a set of goals, it's not enough. They still get distracted, disheartened when anything goes wrong, and bail.

The idea of death, however, can wake you up to how vital those goals are. Death can happen at any point, so learn to appreciate and embrace the *now* in life. If you can do that, I guarantee you will care more about your health, your family, and your children. If I die tomorrow, I know there will be no regrets because

I now care about every moment, every breath of air on this earth, every second I spend with my loved ones—and I try to live life to the best of my ability every day.

You've surely noticed that people who survive a near-death experience suddenly treat life as a gift—for that's what it is, of course. Don't be the person who must endure such a horrific event in order to again appreciate what you have and to remind you what you should be doing with your time on earth.

I had two close friends who had cancer; one died and the other didn't. They both taught me a similar lesson to the one Grandpa did: life is short. You can let such examples go over your head, or get busy and make the most of what you have. After all, what are people going to say after you die? What will you be known for doing? How will your children and grandchildren talk about you? Leave your mark, one that is equally indelible and benefiting for all.

Sometimes we feel half-dead from the pressures of life and simply wish all the crap—weight gain, job difficulties, money problems, sickness, dysfunctional families—would go away as soon as our head hits the pillow. We want to escape into sleep, to vacation, to a stress-free life. Well, I'm asking you to awaken, fully, from such a state and face these challenges head-on. Fortified by Hyperfitness, you will be able to tackle these problems rather than let them overwhelm you. You will improve your life in all categories—you'll get into amazing shape, reduce your stress, and more. And maybe for the first time ever, you won't need a vacation from your own life—you won't want one!

In order to enhance that feeling, **repeat the self-discovery journey** at least twice a year until the day you die. To really feel alive and keep your life progressing, neither you nor your goals should ever stay the same. Keep honing, expanding, and adding—then you will be assured of reaching your potential at every stage of your life.

There are no shortcuts in life. You may have millionaire status but be spiritually bankrupt; you may have built a wonderful family but face enormous financial struggles; you may look better than most cover models, or even be one, but be lonely as hell. These are all examples of people who "invested" and planned for certain areas of their life pretty well, but never addressed other vital areas and are now paying the price. Success is not defined by how much money you have in the bank, but in your soul; your beauty is not the reflection of the mirror, but the love that you give to others. You can avoid such massive gaps by taking a repeated, comprehensive look at your life and where it's headed. Good and bad things don't just happen to you; *you* set them in motion.

Before I headed out upon my own Hyperfitness journey, I had a very conventional view of money and material possessions, as in the more, the better. I wish I could say I wanted more money so I could do more good. Nope, it was all for number one, for I hadn't even met my wife yet. In America, society spends so much time emphasizing the rich life and the way bigger is better, from cars to homes to bank accounts—and I fell for it, hook, line, and sinker.

Each step in my Hyperfitness journey, however, I learned more about myself as a person, and started to want to be in nature more often, meet people from different backgrounds, and promote ideas about environmental sustainability. All the while, my material wealth decreased, yet I was at peace. Now I don't measure success by my bank balance. Happiness and fulfillment didn't come from money, but my internal balance and harmony with life and the people around me.

The Inspiration of Children

SECRET SUMMIT TIP

Children inspired Hyperfitness, and they can inspire you. After all, you were one not *that* long ago. I strongly encourage you to look at the world from a child's perspective. While we adults tend to censor ourselves, children are more like fearless adventurers, always eager to experiment and try new things. Regaining that sense of childlike wonder and invincibility can truly open our lives to the world's never-ending possibilities.

Children walk in truth. Later on they are taught to have prejudices, to lie, to eat poorly, to be inactive. Unspoiled, however, their creative brains can simply amaze and they can be happy with the smallest things. We once did crazy, exciting things as children without thinking it over a dozen times; we lived impetuously, minute to minute, and didn't conform to conventional wisdom. Our imaginations would run wild and little was required to achieve happiness. Let's get that great stuff back.

You will see that many of the exercises, like frog jumping, are ones that children will love doing as well. That's no accident, for a child's movements are spontaneous, magical, and unusual, and so are my workouts. Without necessarily being aware of it, children also essentially do interval training—bursts of activity followed by short rests—and that describes most of my workouts as well. They know what they're doing! They also love natural exercise, and it shows.

This two-chapter prelude to the workouts and nutrition advice in this book may perplex you, as it's unusual for a fitness book. But I've done so because developing a Hypermind is the most important of the three components you need to succeed in this program. Get your mind right, and there are no limits. If I had just handed you a workout and menu plan out of the gate, you wouldn't have had the time to build incentives and prepare mentally for the journey ahead. These first two chapters give you that chance.

Life Is a Circle, Not a Box

Do you compartmentalize the different areas of your life (work, home, vacation, exercise, friends), rather than trying to connect them all? Life is a continuous circle of learning, and each and every action we take matters. As we work toward both our short-term goals and our Inner Everest, it's important for all of us to recognize the valuable links between all aspects of our lives and to create our own circle in which to enjoy the journey.

The world is round, and nature is open for business. In nature, every experience is different, just as every climb I've made up a mountain has been radically different. What I love most about mountains is that they don't care if you're rich or poor, or what clothes you wear—they treat everybody the same and are clearly the great equalizer.

So many of us get caught up in our daily routines, in the pressures of advancing our careers or in the demands of raising a family. We know we are not fulfilling our true mental and physical potential, yet we never seem to find enough time or the right path to get our minds and bodies to where we know they can be. There are so many roles to play in life, but you don't have to play those roles if you're not happy with them. You can be different, more true to yourself, and consequently far happier and more likely to approach your dreams. Living your life in a circle means finding the love in your job, your relationships, in your food and exercise, in how you deal with the outer world. It's about being happy with less, finding that sense of place in your surroundings.

At the base camp of Everest, the Sherpas taught me a lesson that I will never

Ann H., Thirty-six, Elementary School Teacher

"**M**y original workout routine was humdrum to say the least. Everyone has a story for why they can't make it to the gym, and I am no different . . . I attended a variety of exercise classes, and even hired a personal trainer. None of these endeavors were going to keep me coming back to the gym and make exercise a permanent part of my lifestyle. I needed a program that would truly motivate me to work my hardest to achieve my potential.

"The Hyperfitness program has made a huge impact on my life. I feel better today than I did a decade ago. Sean has high expectations and encourages us to achieve our goals both in and out of the gym. He is with us every step of the way on our road to wellness and personally puts his methods to the test, as demonstrated by his impressive running and mountaineering feats. How inspiring to have your instructor 'walk the walk' or in this case, 'run the run.'

"I have been participating in Sean's program before, during, and after pregnancy. To continue with the Hyperfitness program during my pregnancy was the best decision I ever made. A few modifications to the program were required, but the expectations stayed the same. I felt great throughout the entire nine months and was able to continue my workouts until my due date. After the baby, I took a few weeks off, then jumped right back into the Hyperfitness program. Gradually I have achieved, even surpassed, my pre-pregnancy fitness. I have more energy throughout the day, carry less stress with me, and am happier than I've ever been. I am currently looking forward to my first triathlon, something I would have never attempted a few years ago, let alone a few months after having a baby."

forget. I was with a group of Westerners who shared the same climbing permit; we were sitting there, eating in total silence. Meanwhile, I could hear the Sherpas, who were having their meals in a separate tent, laughing and telling stories. They live with next to nothing, some making an average of $220 a year, but they are happy. Sherpas are some of the warmest, most gentle people I've ever known. Rather than derive pleasure from technology, material items, and status, they celebrate the simple things in life: community, fellowship, food, children, and, of course, the mountain. "Wait a minute," we Westerners decry, "I've got the big house and the pool in the backyard and digital cable. Why can't I smile and laugh like that?" Well, if you're not already, you will be soon with this program. You may begin to live a whole new life again.

Chapter 3

ADAPT TO CHANGE

Weeks 1 and 2

O N ONE OF MY TRAINING EXPEDI-
tions before Everest, I climbed Tibet's Shishapangma—one of the highest mountains in the world. When I stood on the summit at almost 26,500 feet, I didn't care that it was 8:30 in the evening or that my climbing partner and I had just broken the most fundamental rule of high-altitude mountaineering survival: If you haven't reached the summit of a high-altitude peak by mid-afternoon, it's probably best to turn around. There is good reason for this rule—it ensures that you'll be climbing back to high camp in daylight hours.

But I had a good reason for my foolishness: I was in love. Venturing out to the surfboard-size summit that showcased a magnificent sunset, I surprised my climbing partner by pulling out an enormous banner from my Himalayan down suit and asking him to take a picture of me. The banner announced "Will you marry me?" (No, I wasn't in love with my climbing partner!) Rather, I was proposing to my girlfriend back in Virginia, who had supported me through all of my climbs and other challenges that life has thrown my way.

My climbing partner, Dan Mazur (one of the finest high-altitude mountaineers in the world, who, in 2006, became famed for saving another climber's life on Everest) was hypoxic, which is like being drunk from lack of oxygen. So he didn't blink at the request and snapped the picture. Holding up the banner in the blustery wind and fighting to not fall over the peak's side, I was a happy man.

My "summit fever," however, was short-lived. Dan and I had chosen the risks associated with descending at night, but I now was psychologically and physically exhausted; my blood was also thickening like maple syrup as a result of the lack of oxygen. I had to adapt in the frozen darkness to weather changes that only intensified my fatigue.

I had wanted to be sure that I could handle the high altitude and grueling nature of Everest, and Shishapangma—known in Tibetan as "the mountain over the grassy plain" and the only 8,000-meter peak wholly in Tibet—was the perfect final test before Everest. True to its reputation, "Shish" had been brutal at times, but this night was something altogether more challenging.

My climbing partner was top-notch, but he, too, was struggling with fatigue and oxygen deprivation. We looked at each other just before the sun said goodbye for the night and, practically at the same time, uttered, "We've got to make it down."

Windy as hell, pitch-black, and freezing cold, the extreme conditions forced me to rely upon all my training. Never did I know how invaluable all the Hyperstrength drills and Inner Everest exercises would be until that point, when I was able to summon a level of strength and determination that I didn't even know I had. Most of all, my Hypermind was ready and willing to do whatever it took to get to high camp. I was not going to let myself get defeated by simply keeping my body churning down the mountain.

By the time we arrived at high camp, it was past 2:30 in the morning and I was shaking from the beginning stages of hypothermia. We could feel the fluid building in our lungs—called pulmonary edema—and knew we'd die unless we got warmed up, fast. We certainly couldn't get any help, as we were two days from the nearest camp. So we set up the stove in our tent as quickly as one can in such a state and got the hot water going. I burned my throat chugging down a cup of extremely hot water, but it still felt good. Right then I knew we'd make it down the mountain alive.

Your willingness to change what you're doing now to embark on this fitness program will make an enormous difference in your body and, moreover, your life. Change only occurs when you leave your comfort zone, so do not let doubt, distractions, or negative influences get in your way.

I am now your climbing partner. I cannot make the climb or produce the sweat for you, but I can show you the trail to the summit. I am giving you the way. You can do this.

Hyperstrength: The New Game in Town

These groundbreaking Hyperstrength workouts were directly inspired by my Everest quest. When I got back to level ground, I knew that I wanted to do a lot more than change people's bodies: I wanted to change their minds about fitness. I was intent on creating workouts that would be challenging to the body and stimulating to the mind—intense, yes, but fun.

Many people train their bodies in a box. They do Pilates or yoga; they take a spin class and do some weights; they spend most of their time lifting, with a little bit of cardio; or they run or cycle, and that's it. There's nothing wrong per se with any of these activities, but so much is left out when you're practicing just one or two of them. While many programs claim to give you a "total body" workout, this is often misleading. They don't actually prepare the body for the many ways it needs to operate in life and sports: fast/slow, power/endurance, fast-twitch/slow-twitch, multiplane, concentric/eccentric/isometric, forward/backward/sideway, running/jumping/shuffling/hopping, and so on.

I want to see you train in a circle so your exercise becomes whole, inclusive, truly total-body, and life-readying. Work to become the complete athlete who can play two hours of tennis, go mountain biking, run a marathon, and play with the kids in the backyard. You don't have to throw out your current workout preferences, such as yoga or cycling. Instead, put them in their proper place, as a complement to a program that does it all for your body: Hyperstrength.

You have your Inner Everest and short-term goal, and you probably have many other active things that you want to do or may just be dreaming about—

maybe playing in a sports league, competing in an endurance event, going on a mountain climb, or taking up a new sport. Or you may simply want to be able to sprint from a train platform, then dash five blocks while carrying a heavy brief-case, and run up six flights of stairs as the elevator is taking way too long get-ting there—because you have exactly seven minutes before you absolutely have to be at work—and arrive cool, smiling, and breathing normally.

My training is unique in that it will prepare you for all of those things—it covers all the bases. You'll find that not only can you play sports such as soc-cer or basketball that you haven't tried since high school, but you can also compete at a very high level for your age group, and even a younger age group. Of course you'll have to practice the skills needed for those specific sports or disciplines in order to improve, but your level of fitness and overall athleticism will already be there. I won the North Pole Marathon by spending most of my training time on Hyperstrength workouts. With my program, you, too, will be able to finish a marathon, for example, without having to log so many hours and pound the road for so many miles. I've had multiple clients who've seen their performance in tennis, golf, basketball, and other sports improve dra-matically after they started doing these workouts, even without specifically working on their games.

Why This Program Works

There are many scientific, physiological reasons why the Hyperstrength drills work so well, but essentially it boils down to four things:

1. improved lactate threshold
2. joint preparedness
3. total muscle fiber stimulation
4. varied training stimulus

(In case you're wondering, you'll also torch tons of calories and get as lean as you've ever wanted to be.) It might sound confusing, but it's really not.

First, lactate, which is lactic acid, is produced in the muscle through duration and intensity of exercise. At some point, the lactic acid reaches a certain level and the muscles begin to shut down; that point is your lactate threshold. Your lactate threshold is also affected by your intake of calories during a workout, a concern for particularly athletic workouts or events lasting longer than an hour. When a cyclist "cracks" during a mountain stage, for example, it is often the result of lactic acid buildup; no matter how mentally strong they are, they can't move their muscles any faster for the remainder of the stage. In these workouts, you'll train hard and fast with short recovery periods, so you'll be building up your body's ability to handle the lactic acid buildup and up your overall threshold. This not only improves your performance levels, but also helps you burn more calories and strengthen your muscle fibers.

Second, your joints will get stimulated from every angle and enjoy a full range of movement, and also get strengthened through plyometric/explosive work. Unlike the pounding nature of some cardiovascular programs, especially running,

Pros and Cons of Running

Running is the number one cardiovascular option for most people, and it's a valuable one, no doubt. In the next chapter, I explain some ways to make your running even more effective.

However, for a few reasons I think it's a mistake to rely solely on running to get fit. First of all, most people run on hard surfaces, which results in joint pounding. Second, because the stress on your joints is approximately two and a half times your weight when you run—which is not true for such workouts as cycling or swimming—if you're carrying any extra pounds, it means even greater stress. Third, a surprising majority of runners may have poor form without knowing it, and this, along with daily repetitive running, can result in various injuries like shin splints, runner's knee, low-back pain, and patellar tendinitis.

Instead, look at one of America's best milers, Alan Webb, who spends 50 percent of his time cross-training. Hyperstrength is cross-training to the nth degree, because you're working your body in as many different ways as possible within a given time frame. For my North Pole marathon, my run training consisted of no more than 30-minute sessions on a treadmill, three times a week, for one month before the race. The cross-training elements within the different Hyperstrength phases, though, was a different story altogether. I never grew tired of the various workouts, and that made all the difference in my preparation for winning the marathon.

that take a toll on your joints, this program will get your joints more resilient than ever. I've had clients with surgically repaired knees who never felt better or more agile. This benefit will come in handy in whatever sport or activity you enjoy, so your joints can more easily handle whatever you put them through.

Third, this workout program will hit all your muscle fibers in every way possible. Through quick, explosive movements and other drills that require more endurance, all of your fast-twitch and slow-twitch muscle fibers will be activated and strengthened—including your ligaments, which lend you even more strength and protect you from injury. Most other programs do only one or the other, so you usually wind up without the coveted results in appearance or performance reality. With Hyperstrength, you'll reap the body-shaping results of fast-twitch training (just like a sprinter gets that enviable physique by employing mostly fast-twitch fibers, which have the greatest capacity to grow) as well as improved overall explosiveness, quickness, speed, and endurance. In addition, your core will be worked in a majority of the moves, so you won't need the overhyped and excessive ab routines that other programs promote.

Fourth, and perhaps most important of all, neither your body nor your mind will ever get stale or bored. The individual workouts are not only unlike any other program you've tried or read about, they also involve a huge variety of moves, many of which involve 360-degree movement. Rather than relying on traditional exercises, over the last ten years I've put a considerable amount of thought into developing innovative moves that deliver the goods. Then, every two weeks, you get treated to brand-new workouts so your mind and muscles can adapt to the next challenges after having conquered the previous weeks'.

In essence, you get the ultimate athletic package with Hyperstrength, which will allow you to improve both your aerobic endurance and anaerobic strength. What does that mean? Developing better aerobic endurance will help you in all these categories: blood flow, slow-twitch muscle fiber strength, heart strengthening, and glycogen storage (the energy within the muscle). Greater anaerobic strength extends to enhanced fast-twitch fibers, lactate threshold, heart rate stroke volume, and VO_2 (see page 268) max—all of which are a very big deal if you want to be an athlete, compete as an athlete, or just live a long time!

I'm going to make you the athlete you always wanted to be or were before. You know what—I'm going to make you an even better athlete!

The Techniques of Hyperstrength Success

You're probably starting to get it about now—get what Hyperfitness is about, and, in this chapter, what Hyperstrength involves. I want to share with you a little more about why it works, and what kind of training you'll be doing.

A key element of the Hyperstrength program is keeping your body guessing with each exercise day. At the health club and at home many people do similar workouts every time, with the same weights, the same cardiovascular equip-

---

"New School Strength" Versus "Old School Strength"

Many of the current exercise routines that involve weights are "old school." I use the term "old school" to describe the dominant influence bodybuilding has on strength training, including the tendency to isolate muscle groups, take long rests between sets, and work only part of the body on given days. There is one purpose and one purpose only: to build more muscle, or mass.

Unfortunately, nearly every exercise machine has the same limitations (the one big exception is the cable machines that force you to stabilize on the floor with your own feet). They isolate a particular muscle group on your body and require little to no ability to balance the weight. In other words, they may make your muscles bigger—but only the obvious ones and not the smaller or harder-to-hit muscles, which causes an imbalanced physique and a risk of injury. In other words, machines don't promote real, functional strength that benefits you in sports, or life. (The other reason there are so many machines, for every muscle in the body, and so many manufacturers? To make money, of course.)

If you're being trained or have been trained by a personal trainer who's put you on a split program (working different muscles on different days) and takes you around to these different isolating machines, then you are/were on a bodybuilding program, whether you know it or not. Did I hear a few screams?

You may knowingly be on such a program right now. But are you getting the results you want? If you're aiming to look like a bodybuilder, great, stick with the big weights, machines, and isolation routine.

But if you want to be an athlete who can move quickly and endure activity for sustained periods of time; if you want to possess real strength that can work for you no matter what task or sport you do; then please follow the Hyperstrength way. Be like Bruce Lee, who was only a buck thirty but had a one-inch punch that could knock you back six feet because his ligaments and fibers were so strong. Now that's new-school strength.

ment, for the same length of time. These people never seem to be getting in better shape, and in many cases their bodies decline in fitness and looks. Their bodies have become efficient in their exercise routine, so they consume fewer calories. Joggers, for instance, who always run about the same distance at roughly the same speed expend fewer and fewer calories as time goes on. Their bodies are programmed to know what to do because they have adapted to the stresses; their bodies will no longer produce larger muscles or burn a greater amount of fat because they're more efficient in executing the workout. The progression has ended, and only a decline can result.

In Hyperfitness, I'll give at least two very different workouts over a two-week time period, and then shift to two brand-new workouts for the next two weeks. Every workout is total body, with hardly any isolation moves. The goal is simple: to engage as many muscle groups as you possibly can, in as many ways as you can, in a fixed time frame. Your legs, for example, have a tremendous reservoir of power and endurance, but few training programs tap into this reservoir properly; they either underwork them (such as in a typical bodybuilding program that hits the quads only once or twice a week) or they overwork them, often by means of a repetitive movement like running, sometimes resulting in repetitive stress injuries. In Hyperstrength, you'll use your legs a lot, but in drastically different ways—and they will carry you farther than you've ever imagined.

One of the most frequent moves in the Hyperstrength workout is the squat, of which I give many variations. It's one of our most natural movements in sports and life in general, yet so few programs really capitalize on its potential for hitting a maximum number of muscle fibers in the legs as well as building cardiovascular and muscular strength. Similarly, the push-up is the upper body's squat, because it uses so many different muscle groups and allows you to employ many different variations.

You will work all of your muscles, some more than others on particular days, for five or six days a week, because that is how real athletes train. That line about how "each muscle group needs forty-eight hours of recovery" is a fabrication from the bodybuilding world, not from the real one. Bodybuilders do require that kind of recovery time because they absolutely blitz each of their muscle groups with weights; they're on a search for muscle size, not muscle utility. You're not going to be doing chest and biceps, then call it a day; you're also not going to work out just two or three times a week and expect to see big-time benefits. Look at top-level athletes like LeBron James, Steve House, and Maria Sharapova—they look great and perform at insanely high levels because they're using all of their muscles almost every day.

Even if you belong to the most state-of-the-art gym in the world, I want you to forgo the shiny weight machines and stick with dumbbells, physioballs, pull-up bars, medicine balls, cable machines, and the like. Using these types of equipment allows you to employ multijoint movements and use a greater range of motion, which results in greater strength, muscle involvement, athleticism, flexibility, and calorie burn.

If you exercise at home, you can get in a terrific Hyperstrength workout using dumbbells alone (as well as just your own body weight in many moves), especially when combined with a stability ball. Dumbbells help you develop real-world, functional strength movements such as pushing, pulling, squatting, rotating, stepping, and jumping. Essentially they duplicate how you would lift loads in everyday life, and they sculpt a symmetrical physique in which both arms and legs are of equal strength (most machines don't account for the fact that one side of your body holds more than 50 percent of the load and, inevitably, you wind up with muscle imbalance). What's more, dumbbells also "recruit" many more muscle fibers surrounding the targeted muscle groups—such as the invaluable stabilizer muscles around joints like the shoulder, elbow, hips, knees, and ankles.

All the moves in Hyperstrength are functional first, rather than cosmetic. You will end up looking a lot leaner and stronger every week that goes by, rather than doing moves that won't do much beyond making your biceps look better. You will perform multiplane movements to develop a complete strength and complete athleticism that you have never experienced before. Some of these functional drills will literally throw you off-balance, but what they are designed to do is build your balance, agility, stability, and coordination.

Many of the drills are based on the principles of plyometrics. They are de-

Gearing Up for Hyperstrength

Many of the Hyperstrength moves will only require your body weight, but at minimum I would like you to have a few **dumbbells,** a **medicine ball,** a **stability ball,** a **mat,** and a **jump rope** at your disposal—and a solid pair of **trail-running shoes.** Beyond dumbbells, which we discussed earlier, this other equipment is vital to the program as well. A stability ball helps engage your core in almost every move and also improves your balance. A medicine ball assists with the multiplane, 360-degree movements within your exercises. A mat removes discomfort when you do any floor exercise. A jump rope delivers both plyometric and cardiovascular benefits at the same time, and is fun to use. Trail-runners allow you to move in any direction, including squatting, jumping, and running, both safely and soundly.

Dumbbells: beginners (Trekkers) should purchase two of the following poundages: 5, 10, 15, 20, and 25. Or, if you're coming from a completely sedentary background, go with this combination: 3, 5, 8, 12, and 15. For intermediate (Climbers) and advanced (Sherpas) students, your dumbbell weights should go higher by five-pound increments. Your rack could look like this: 5, 10, 15, 20, 25, 30, 35, 40, 45, 50, 55, and 60. Though you may choose to wait until you can more easily handle heavier dumbbells to purchase any dumbbells above 40 pounds.

Medicine balls: The weight of your medicine balls will depend upon your fitness level. My suggestion is to purchase just one ball, anywhere from a 4- to 8-pounder, that will challenge you for the first four weeks. As you get stronger, purchase heavier medicine balls.

Stability ball: It must be the right size for your height, so when you sit on the middle of the ball your thighs are parallel to the ground. Generally, the more expensive the stability ball, the better the quality.

Mat: Standard exercise mats, yoga mats, and Pilates mats are the most common mats sold. All will suffice, but some many prefer the Pilates mats because of superior thickness and quality.

Jump rope: Almost any jump rope will do the job, but ropes with ball bearings operate the most smoothly. On the other hand, ropes made of genuine rope don't hold up very well.

Trail-running shoes: Aim to purchase a trail-running shoe that fits both the length of your foot and width. Depending on the climate in which you exercise, consider waterproof and/or insulated varieties.

If you belong to a well-equipped gym or want to outfit your own home gym further, then you will be able to take advantage of even more Hyperstrength moves

signed to throw you for a loop, especially in the beginning, but they are an amazing conditioning technique. They build your power, which is primarily housed in your fast-twitch muscle fibers. Plyometric drills allow you to activate the largest amounts of your muscle fibers because you are generating your highest and combinations. I recommend that you begin with the above equipment and, if you're committed to this program, you can invest further into some or all of the following equipment. After all, you're building a new and improved you—and none of this equipment will cost you too much. Here is some recommended *extra Hyperstrength Equipment.*

Treadmill: Owning a treadmill is very convenient when weather is prohibitive to outdoor exercise. It also allows you to exercise right next to the rest of your exercise equipment, so you're able to intermix exercises and drills (which we do a lot in Hyperstrength!) without difficulty.

Stationary bike: A stationary bike is equally practical and may be the way to go for overweight individuals who want to reduce the weight-bearing activity at the beginning of the program. Owning a bike in addition to a treadmill gives you another great cardio option for the program, and some training days are tailored for the bike rather than the treadmill.

Weighted jump rope: In addition to a regular rope, purchase a 1-pound, 2-pound, 3-pound, and 4-pound rope, which I call "weighted cables." As you improve your fitness level, you can move up in rope poundage.

Bosu: Like a stability ball, the Bosu engages your muscles to stabilize your body. This time you're standing or your hands are on the piece of equipment.

Heart rate monitor: This gives you feedback on how hard you are exercising, so you're less likely to overtrain or undertrain. But do not come to depend on one. I rarely use mine anymore and prefer to listen to my own body for the monitoring of intensity and performance levels.

Plyometric box or step: You can purchase plyometric (plyo) boxes—or, more cheaply, a step with additional risers—or you can build one yourself with two-by-fours and plywood. The platform on top of your box should measure about 24 inches by 24 inches.

Rings/straps: Rings and/or straps are essential pieces of equipment for Climbers and Sherpas, and for helping create real-life strength because they enhance body-weight exercises.

Bands: Bands are convenient to use when traveling.

Kettlebell: This cowbell-shaped weight with a handle is an excellent alternative to dumbbells and medicine balls. Begin with a 20- to 30-pound kettlebell.

See Appendix F for recommended suppliers.

power output with each explosive rep. Plyometrics will not only make you a better athlete, or an athlete for the first time in your life, but they will also serve you down the road. Your fast-twitch fibers are the first muscle fibers to erode as you age unless you train them. These are the muscles developed in the healthy, strong-looking older adult who not only carries an impressive musculature but also is much less prone to falls because his or her agility remains intact.

You're also never going to sit down during our sessions together, unless it's on the stability ball or at the end of a workout. (By the way, the fact that more than half of the machines offer you a seat, and a padded leather one at that, is indicative of how ineffective modern gym training is today—this is supposed to be about breaking a sweat, not going first class on a plane!) Again, you want to activate as many muscles as possible, and standing, or sitting on a stability ball, accomplishes that. And it allows you to operate in three planes of motion and to burn up to 50 percent more calories than if you were seated.

Remember when I talked about how the Hyperstrength workout gives you aerobic endurance and anaerobic strength in one package? The Inner Everest (IE) drills are specifically designed to build both by doing different exercises consecutively without rest. The IE drills will trick your mind, meaning that your brain will think it's getting a break by doing something new, but the exercises will still be challenging your aerobic endurance while working a different part of your body anaerobically. This type of training is far more effective than just running or cycling habitually. Plus I add mantra, visualization, and breathing techniques within the IE drills to top off the effectiveness of the exercises and to build your Hypermind intensity (more on this later).

You will keep your body so busy during these workouts that you will forget how fatigued you might be. Your body will acclimate to the high intensity, not focusing on the discomfort; instead, the effort will exhilarate you. Meanwhile, your body will get leaner and your heart will work better. It's the opposite of the typical workout in which you're just waiting for the time to go by. Here it will fly, and you will be in the moment. And after you finish, you will have a glow that you carry with you the rest of the day.

Where You're At—*Now*

At this point, you will select your training level for the Hyperstrength program. Are you a Trekker, who is relatively out of shape and starting this program after either exercising only infrequently, a long layoff, or living a previously sedentary life? Or are you a Climber, who has been working out and training for a while, and is ready for something more arduous that will get you to the next level? You might even be a Sherpa, who is already in great shape, may be an accomplished athlete, and is ready for something new and challenging.

Before you answer, you need to evaluate carefully which level suits you. It is critically important to accurately and unflinchingly evaluate your level. Choosing a level too hard for you may not only cause burnout, it can cause injury as well. You may overreach in the beginning and find you need to build more gradually, or you may be surprised to learn that you are capable of more than you had previously imagined. Don't sweat the decision too much, for I will provide body checks to make sure you've selected the appropriate level for you. (IMPORTANT: It is essential that you see a doctor for a full physical check-up before beginning the Hyperstrength phase of this program, or any type of physical program.)

The following questions will determine your level, but only if you are completely honest with your answers. Don't worry if you start at the Trekker level—it will definitely challenge you. If you are dead set on getting to the Sherpa level one day, you will—don't worry. For each question, write down the appropriate number of points that correspond to your answer, and add up the total at the end.

Remember, the levels given here are only suggestions. If you are having an extremely difficult time getting through the first day in any of the levels, I suggest you start at the Trekker level. This level is suitable for all types of athletes and nonathletes and will help establish a good foundation for your program.

It's crucial that you start off slowly, so I'd like you to complete a self-evaluation to determine your aerobic ceiling heart rate (see Appendix E), which, used in conjunction with the Hyperfitness Exertion Scale (H.E.S.), will inform you of the exertion levels you are exercising at in your current level.

You've built up your mind, refined your goals, and are ready for the physical challenge. But I want you to have patience with yourself and with the program. There may be moments and days where you want to bail or get frustrated, so have faith that you can do this. It may physically challenge you more than you have ever been challenged before, so don't be too hard on yourself if you don't complete an exercise or miss a workout. Just get back on the horse if you want to ride to your goals. I knew that if I rushed too quickly and tried to climb Everest in a short period of time, the shock alone from the immediate extreme change would have pushed me in the opposite direction and my goals would never have been realized.

In the next twelve weeks, you will build a solid, strong base. These programs

QUESTION	1 POINT	2 POINTS	3 POINTS	4 POINTS	
How many days do you exercise per week?	5–7	3–4	2–1	0	
How many days a week do you exercise with weights, including both upper and lower body?	5–7	3–4	2–1	0	
How fast can you run an average mile?	Under 7 minutes	Under 8 minutes	Under 9 minutes	Over 9 minutes	
When was the last time you exercised on a regular, consistent basis?	I do now	A few months ago	A long time ago	Never	
What grade do you give yourself for daily activity?	Excellent	Good	Average	Poor	
What is the overall intensity of your exercising? Small, moderate, large, or no increase in pulse and/or breathing?	Large	Moderate	Small	None	
How long is your average workout?	Over 1½ hours	1 hour	Under 1 hour	Not at all	
How do you feel about exercising?	Enjoy	Ups and downs	Don't like	Hate	
Do you have any illness or medical problems?	None	Mild	Moderate	Severe	

POINT TOTALS:

21 to 36 = **Trekker**
13 to 20 = **Climber**
12 and under = **Sherpa**

were meticulously designed to become increasingly challenging, so there's no need to push too much too soon.

Don't Forget the Goal!

Before you jump into the program, take this opportunity to go over your goals one more time. I trust that you've identified your Inner Everest goal. Now let's make sure you've got a reasonable short-term goal for the twelve-week Hyperstrength program and that it works for your current fitness level.

Experience has taught me that a physical regimen is more rewarding when one has a purpose and clear results to strive for, so double-check that your goal is both inspiring and attainable. Perhaps you're wavering about which one to go with. If so, here are some options:

Trekker: Do an 8K race, hike up a small mountain, take an active vacation with your family, join a sports league, pick up a new sport, start commuting to work by bicycle.

Climber: Do a half or full marathon, take an all-day hike, sprint a distance triathlon, do a first-time adventure race, take a mountaineering course, take a mountain bike course, do a century bike race, take an extended canoeing trip.

Sherpa: Do a 50K race, climb a high or technical mountain, do a full Ironman.

These are all first-rate goals, as long as they are challenging, new to the senses, and they help you continue to take steps forward on the path of a goal-oriented fitness lifestyle.

If one of the goals you are intent on accomplishing requires a specific set of skills, then first complete twelve weeks of Hyperstrength training to give you a great base to operate from. Then spend a few weeks working on the specific skills that you will need, and continue doing the Hyperstrength workouts until you're ready. To assist you in reaching those goals, keep a **training log** of your progress that records such things as which exercises you struggle with and which ones you don't, your heart rate levels, and the time it takes to finish the workouts.

My first short-term goal was to take on a short, three-day technical "clinic" by climbing Mount Rainier in Washington. From my knowledge and background reading, I knew that Rainier would be a perfect starting point because the mountain contained all the hazards of Everest—crevasses, wind, and weather—but without the high altitude.

The Countdown . . .

There's just a little more ground I want to cover before you begin your week-one workout. First, there's the matter of **when to work out.** I'm going to ask you to create time for your exercising, rather than trying to find the time to work out or attempting to "squeeze in a workout." Put those five or six weekly workouts, depending on your level, into your calendar/daily planner and maybe your cell phone/Blackberry/Treo in advance.

For most people, the best time to work out is in the morning, about an hour after waking up. If you are not a morning person, try to become one; it may make or break the program for you. Too often the decision to exercise in the afternoon or evening gets pushed to the side because a meeting went late, work took longer than you had planned, or you had family matters to deal with. I've seen it with countless people: Those who work out in the morning rarely miss their sessions.

That being said, if the morning slot just doesn't work for you and your schedule, try to stick to another regular time of day to exercise. Your body comes to expect activity at a certain time of day after a while, so the transition from everyday activity to Hyperstrength activity will be a smoother one. In the beginning, if you're unaccustomed to training after work, for instance, you may find yourself flagging.

Hyperfare: Workout Foods and Liquids

No matter what time of day you exercise, it's important for you to get a blood sugar boost before beginning the workout; preworkout nutrition will not only allow you to complete the workout more easily, it will also help increase your overall performance and calorie expenditure.

For the morning movers, have a preworkout light meal of about 60 to 120 calories approximately twenty to thirty minutes before exercising. A slice of whole-grain toast, a banana, or some organic yogurt will do nicely. If you work out a couple of hours after getting up, then make sure you consume a full breakfast. Then before the workout have something light just to get the blood sugar up again, like half a banana or half a piece of toast with a little peanut butter. If you start later in the day, follow the same nutrition design, making sure you wait at least two hours after a full meal and consume something light twenty to thirty minutes prior to the session.

The best ratio of carbohydrates to protein for the preworkout meal is 4 to 1. Do your best to avoid the workout drinks and bars, because many contain processed sugars and they possess far more calories than you need. Only if you're training for more than an hour will you need such calorie loads. And whatever you do, don't train on an empty stomach, especially first thing in the morning, because you'll not only run out of gas during the workout but set yourself up for gorging later in the day. Treat your body with respect and it will respond accordingly. Just like a kid who doesn't behave very well if he doesn't get his snacks and meals on time, you, too, need to take in good calories at key times before and after workouts.

It's also key to walk into the workouts well hydrated. During the workouts that last under an hour, take in only water. If you feel nauseated while exercising, it may be because you are showing signs of dehydration. If you go for more than an hour, especially on a hot day, I recommend a small electrolyte-replacement drink of no more than 120 calories, or an energy gel. If you exercise for at least ninety minutes on a hot day, take a sodium tablet for salt loss from sweat secretion. I follow a simple guide to hydration that has never failed me—I drink when I am thirsty.

After exercise, your body needs nutrients during the "glycogen window," in which your muscles require refilling of valuable glycogen for faster muscle recovery, less soreness, and better energy levels afterward. How big is that window? Well, ideally, you should take in at least 100 to 150 calories of nutrition (again, the 4 to 1 ratio) within twenty to forty-five minutes after finishing. Within ninety minutes after the workout or event, eat a full meal of healthy carbohydrates, protein, and fiber, as well as some essential fats. The carbohydrates replenish your muscle glycogen stores, and the protein assists the repair of damaged muscle tissue. Again, energy bars or meal replacement shakes cannot fill the same valuable role of regular healthy meals; they do not contain the nutrients that fruits and quality proteins deliver to your body.

If you are unaccustomed to eating after working out, or don't even feel hungry, well, just eat a good amount anyway. Your body requires those nutrients and calories for improved recovery, metabolic function, and future performance!

Without Further Ado . . . Your Hyperstrength Program

This is it. This initial two-week Hyperstrength phase will emphasize aerobic and strength-foundation building, and you will be asked to focus mainly on bodyweight and dumbbell exercises for daily training, and core exercises to establish solid base levels of fitness. All levels will perform an Inner Everest drill for balance and agility training to establish their current aptitude.

If you've used other training programs before, you will probably notice some major differences right away. First, my **exercises are unique,** as are the combinations that I put together. I'm not saying that all conventional moves are bad news, but I simply believe that unique exercises are far more stimulating for your mind as well as your body; they work for me, and I know they'll work for you.

Second, the **repetitions will be more numerous** than what you've likely experienced before. We are working on building your lactate threshold, so lactic acid in your muscles doesn't shut down your muscles after a certain point. Many of the individual exercises last for at least a minute, and I expect you to make it until that point, because the last 10 percent of those sets is when the benefit truly kicks in.

Third, as we work on lactate-threshold training, we also will be **limiting the**

rests between sets to increase your threshold and improve your overall fitness level. Resting between sets is one of the biggest wastes of time in modern-day workouts, and it actually sabotages your gains! The mark of great athletes is that they can perform at near-peak levels for extended periods of time. This kind of workout, with high-intensity exercises followed by short rests, will build you into the kind of athlete you've always dreamed of becoming.

In addition, reduced rest time causes your body to produce more "physique-enhancing hormones" that alert your body to build muscle and lose fat. In the beginning, you may need to rest more until you get the hang of it and your muscles and lungs adapt, but make it your goal to take fewer and fewer rests.

You will also use **strength combinations:** exercises that you do consecutively, without rest in between. Supersets (doing a set of exercises and then following up with a different set that involves an opposite movement, such as the push/pull exercises) and double-ups (completing an exercise and then immediately doing another exercise using the same muscle groups) are forms of combinations. (Just please don't use the word *circuit* to describe any part of this program, since circuit training is forever linked to machine-based workouts.) Combinations do many things well: They raise your lactate threshold, hit every muscle in your body over the course of several exercises, fool your body into thinking it's getting a rest when it's only actually getting a new exercise, burn a maximum amount of calories, improve your VO_2 max (see page 268), and build greater agility and overall athleticism. Not bad, eh?

You must make sure you use **excellent exercise form** with all the moves. Read the exercise descriptions carefully prior to working out (even the night before), and follow them to a T. The movements are also more dynamic than other exercises, so take your time whenever you're doing a new exercise, especially for the first sets. And with the plyometric/explosive moves, try to restrict your time and contact points with the ground as much as possible, which will enhance fast-twitch muscle development and overall speed.

Even though there are more than 125 photographs to help provide you with correct form, there are more than 300 different drills for the entire program. You

Warm-up for All Levels

Focus on continual movements during the Hyperstrength warm-up. You're working to increase the temperature of your body in order to prime your muscles and joints for the exercises that will follow. The warmup exercises are low impact, should be done in a controlled manner, and should never include locking out any joints.

As in tai chi, follow your body rather than resist it. So when a drill causes you to switch directions, do so fluidly. Allow your body and mind to sync up, and the harmony will boost your workout considerably.

Trekker, Climber, and Sherpa—do 2 rounds:

Standing alternate toe touches—20 reps

Shallow jumping jacks (do not commit to a full range of motion)—20 reps

Body squats (with feet shoulder-width apart, squat down with an erect torso until thighs are almost parallel to ground) with left/right knee lifts—15 reps

Cross taps (Left elbow touches right knee, right elbow touches left knee)—20 reps total

High knee marching (in place or moving forward)—20 reps

may require the Hyperstrength DVD set that visually illustrates each individual exercise for your specific level. (For more information go to www.HyperfitnessLiving.com.)

Last, it's important to **warm up** properly before beginning each day's program. If you warm up properly, it is not necessary to fully stretch (which, in my experience, is more useful *after* the workout).

The Beginning: Weeks 1 and 2

Day 1 of the program is upon you. If you aren't already, get excited! Prepare to get stronger and increasingly fit, day after day, week after week. Open yourself to physical challenges that you've never faced before, and expect to see and feel huge improvements in your body, mind, and even your soul. If you have any previous negative associations with exercise, Hyperstrength will obliterate them. This is the new way of exercising and puts you squarely on the cutting edge.

These workouts will benefit everything you currently do—in your work, family, sport, or leisure—and every goal you have.

Along those lines, here's one last reminder to sign up for a race, organized hike, or some other inner-self, short-term physical test that should be undertaken immediately following the end of the twelve-week program. It will help keep you on track and motivated just as much as your Inner Everest goal. This is where your dreams are so important, for they can provide the fuel for your workouts. Any great athlete is fueled by dreams to be the best in their sport. Maybe simply competing in a sport is your short-term goal, or going on a physical family outing that you've thought about for years. Whatever drives you is what belongs in your set of goals.

Just don't settle for the "lose a few pounds" ambition, for that will take care of itself! Hyperfitness is a lifestyle, and much more than a series of cool workouts. The physical program in this book can change your life if you're committed to more than simply exercising to look better. That is a wonderful short-term goal, but it should not be the essence of why you are changing your life. The weight will come off and the lean muscles will appear, but then what's next? I want that "next" part to be in your mind, *now*.

Why Am I So Sore?

The first two weeks will create soreness in muscles you never even knew you had! This is expected, and it's called Delayed Onset Muscle Soreness (DOMS); it comes from putting your muscles under a strain that they're unaccustomed to, which results in tiny microscopic tears in your muscle fibers and tissues at a cellular level. This is a positive development, because with ample time to recover, your muscles will repair themselves and grow back stronger.

Instead of ceasing or slowing down your exercise, however, it's imperative that you keep up with the program in order to keep the blood flowing to your muscles to help them recover. Along with stretching and Hyperfare nutrition, the Hyperstrength routine eventually will create less soreness as you get more fit.

Learn to love the soreness. Be like the great huskies; we, too, are animals who work, and who are usually most happy when we're physically using our bodies.

SECRET SUMMIT TIP

What to Do with the Weekends

The weekends are the time to let it all go: binge with junk food, beer, and a few margaritas, and don't move a muscle. Ah, yeah, right! I just wanted to make sure you were reading this carefully. The weekend is the perfect time for active cleansing and relaxation. Rather than grinding away at the gym and at work, get outside and do activities that weekends are meant for. Visit a museum with friends or family, take a walk in the park, or have a picnic and take a Frisbee along. Go on a hike in the nearest national park, visit the closest city to you and actually do the tourist attractions, or take a bike ride with your children.

If you have chores around the house to do, stay active rather than zone out in front of the ball game or endless movies. After all, the less you sit around, the less likely you are to make repeated trips to the fridge.

The body and mind need to be revitalized continually, especially after a tough week. An interesting, stimulating weekend will lift your spirits for the coming week. Accordingly, do at least one thing that works toward your goals on the weekend, even if it is something as simple as researching a subject, on the Internet for a half hour, such as an inspirational person who has accomplished the same goal you have set.

In order to keep focused on each workout and make it more efficient, bring in the two-week plan to each training session rather than try to work from memory. Trust me.

TREKKER

The majority of you should undergo the Trekker phase first. You will be working out for thirty to forty-five minutes five days a week. It may seem daunting at first, but in order to build real-life strength and cardiovascular conditioning, you will need to devote this amount of time at a minimum.

This Trekker program will mainly consist of body-weight exercises, with limited free-weight exercises. Some people think that machinery is needed for a productive workout, but I've trained some of the fittest people in the country with nothing but body-weight exercises. You can get a productive workout wherever you choose, for you're not bound by expensive equipment and health club memberships. As long as you follow the illustrations and explanations closely and carefully, you'll cover serious ground to higher fitness levels than you ever thought possible.

Music for Motivation

SECRET SUMMIT TIP

Music can be a powerful tool to increase energy levels, though silence or nature sounds can be equally inspiring. Go with your mood—sometimes music may be just the thing you need to get your blood going and other times your mind desperately needs no distractions except for your training.

The music I personally listen to is wide-ranged. When in doubt, I'll go with hard and aggressive. Others, however, may be just as motivated by a powerful concerto or jazz trio. Studies have shown that on average people work 11 percent harder when they are listening to music they enjoy or that is motivational. Listening to music while you exercise also increases brainpower. Your mind is actively retrieving the beats, rhythm, and sound of the music.

Try to avoid using music as a crutch, however—I will often encourage you to simply take in the outdoors rather than live within your own iPod. And if you're competing in an athletic event, chances are you won't be able to take your tunes with you, so practice training hard without any music at all. Also, once a week, listen to music you dislike during a workout session—train the mind to get into the zone, away from the sounds, singing, and beats. Drown out the sound in your mind by concentrating on every breath you take and each movement of the exercises you are performing.

A Climber and a Trekker

HF TESTIMONIAL

For Glen L., an information technology consultant and father of two who exercises on the Climber level, the goal was to compete in an adventure race. Before he began Hyperfitness, Glen explains, "Competing in multisport races over thirty miles and lasting over seven hours seemed to me the events of single, twenty-something fitness fanatics, human freaks of nature. Hyperfitness led me to be competitive in these adventure races. I've been able to accomplish goals and exceed targets I never could have on my own."

For Debbie D., who works at the National Rural Utilities Cooperative Finance Corporation and exercises on the Trekker level, the goal was to complete the Washington, D.C., AIDS Ride, a 330-mile bicycle ride from Raleigh, North Carolina, to Washington, D.C., which benefits local AIDS charities. "Through the Hyperfitness program I trained for the D.C. AIDS Ride and endured a physically and mentally challenging training schedule for four months. I attribute the will and drive I had while training to the challenges I took on with Sean in his programs."

Hyperstrength Stretches

If you warm up properly, there is really no need to stretch before the workout. That said, I spend about three minutes doing quick, ten-second flex stretching, moving through a few joint manipulative techniques to eliminate any tiny gas bubbles in the joint fluid, limber up any muscles that may be tight, and unbind any locked or pinched joints. (This occurs whenever you hear a crack or pop when making a sudden movement.)

Stretching *after* exercise is what really makes a difference. It helps decrease muscle tightness, reduces muscle fatigue, retains muscle elasticity, and prevents tears and injury. Your aim is to make your ligaments and tendons strong like bamboo, as does a practitioner of Ashtanga yoga. I also use stretching as a way to calm my mind and help regenerate my body mechanics.

Breathe only through your nose, because nasal breathing 1) forces you to focus on the inhalation and exhalation within the movements, and 2) keeps you from holding your breath, as many individuals unknowingly do.

Hold each stretch or pose anywhere from 10 to 30 seconds, 2 to 3 times.

Tibetan Squat: My personal favorite, which I learned in Southeast Asia, it helps with flexibility in the spine, shoulders, knees, ankles, hips, and hamstrings. Go from standing position down into a deep squat with your toes pointed out 45 degrees. Be sure to keep your heels on the floor. Extend both arms forward as if reaching for something just out of reach on the floor. Hold the stretch for 15 seconds. Come up and repeat.

Supine Hamstring Hug: Lying on your back, straighten one leg while bending the other near your chest. Hold your arms as close to the chest as possible. Hold at just below the knee of your bent leg. After 10 seconds, move the hold to your shin and push in for a deeper stretch. After another 10 seconds, hold just above the ankle and bring your leg to your chest for an even deeper stretch.

Wall Calf Stretch: Lean against a wall with one leg in front of the other and both heels on the floor, feet pointed forward. Lean forward until you feel a stretch on your back leg. Alternate by bending your

CLIMBER

To be a Climber, you should feel comfortable exercising on a fairly consistent basis, meaning that you're not unduly sore after most sessions and you rarely miss any workouts. Having mastered the Trekker level, you'll be ready for greater challenges. This program will get you to that next level.

SHERPA

In order for me to be strong enough to climb Everest, I exercised for one and a half hours a day, six days a week, and practiced the physical training of the back knee to stretch the other part of your calf. Repeat on the other side.

Hip Flexor Stretch: Lie on your back, with both knees bent and your feet flat on the floor. Place your right ankle on top of your left knee and lift your left leg off the floor. Interlace your hands behind your left kneecap, bringing your left leg toward your chest and keeping your right leg bent. When you feel the stretch, hold for 30 seconds, then switch sides.

Straddle Stretch: Sitting up, spread your legs wide into a "V." Reach out with your left hand toward your right foot. Hold for 20 seconds, then point your toes out and hold for another 20 seconds. Repeat on the other side.

Prone Shoulder Stretch: Lying facedown on the floor, extend one arm out perpendicular to your body, palm down. Turn in the other direction to face up and roll up so you feel a stretch in your chest and shoulders. Hold for 20 seconds, relax for 5 seconds, then repeat 1 time.

Kneeling Hip Flexor: Kneel with your right leg on the floor and bend your left knee 90 degrees so your left foot is on the floor. Extend your right leg behind you so the top of the foot is on the floor. Place both palms on the floor on either side of your left foot and shift your weight forward until you feel a stretch in your hip. Hold for 20 seconds, then repeat once. Switch to the other leg and repeat.

The Hands-to-Feet Walk: In an inverted "V" position with your heels on the floor and your fingers spread wide on the floor, hold for 10 seconds, then walk your hands back until they meet your toes. Repeat 3 times.

Standing Quadriceps Stretch: Stand, using a wall for balance if needed. Bend your left knee directly behind you and grasp your left ankle with your left hand. Make sure you stand erect while pulling your heel toward your glute. Hold the pose for a count of 20 seconds, then switch to the other leg and repeat.

Hero Pose: Kneel on the floor, keeping your legs hip-width apart. Try to point your toes straight back. Relax your upper body in sitting position while stretching your quadriceps and tibias anteriors (front lower legs). Hold for 30 seconds.

Sherpa level, as well as integrating exercises from the Climber and Trekker levels. Frankly, I would have loved to have trained more, but I had a job that took up the rest of my time. So it works, let me tell you, and it's also very challenging. High-caliber weekend warriors and athletes who are reading this book may choose to start here, but it will push even them to their limits. Those of you who are in great shape but unsure of how to go further, here it is.

TREKKER ▲ Weeks 1 and 2 • Monday/Wednesday/Friday

Go straight through the 6 drills below, 3 times, with a 2 to 3 minute rest between each complete round of exercises. For the dumbbell drills, select a weight—anywhere from 5 to 30 pounds—that will challenge you for 1 minute (you may be surprised at how quickly your muscles fatigue, so in the beginning, underestimate your current strength). If your muscles exhaust before the minute is reached, rest as needed, then continue until 1 minute is up.

1. **Incline Dumbbell Press on Stability Ball**
2. **Downward Jumping Jack to Full Upward Jack**
3. **Staggered Squat to Bent-over Row with Dumbbell**
4. **Squat Jump to 2 Bounces**
5. **Triceps Push-up on Knees to Clap**
6. **Squat to Dumbbell Overhead Press**

IE Drill: Go straight through the 3 drills with little to no rest between them. For each drill, go 15 yards down and back; repeat the round 3 more times, again with as little rest as possible. Hyperfitness exertion scale (H.E.S. 2–3).

1. **Alternate Lunge**
2. **Side-to-Side Squat (with hand swoop)**
3. **Carioca**

Core: Go straight through the 2 exercises with no rest; repeat twice for 15 reps each.

1. **Straight-Leg Crunch**
2. **Oblique Roll-up**

Stretch (see pages 58–59)

Incline Dumbbell Press on Stability Ball: Sit on the ball, with your feet flat on floor, and hold the dumbbells at your sides. Slide your butt down the ball until the ball rests between your shoulder blades and your torso makes a 45-degree angle. From this position, execute a chest press with the dumbbells in a controlled manner.

Downward Jumping Jack to Full Upward Jack: Get into push-up position, with your arms straight and underneath your shoulders. With your upper body holding that position, jump both legs out in spread-eagle fashion so your toes touch out, and then come back to push-up position. Next, jump your feet to under your chest, stand up, and do a full upward jumping jack. Clap your hands overhead and then behind your lower back on the way down.

Staggered Squat to Bent-over Row with Dumbbell: With a dumbbell in your right hand hanging down at your side, assume a boxing stance with your left leg forward and right leg back, knees bent, feet flat on the floor. With an erect torso, squat downward, until your front thigh is almost parallel to the floor. From that position, lean forward slightly (without rounding your back) and pull the dumbbell upward to beside your rib cage as you rise from the squat, feet still in boxing stance. Switch sides after completing the set.

Squat Jump to 2 Bounces: With your arms clasped in front of your chest, squat downward until your thighs are parallel to the ground and your heels remain on the ground. Explode upward, trying to get maximum height. Upon landing, do 2 quick bounces before the next squat jump.

Standard Squat Position

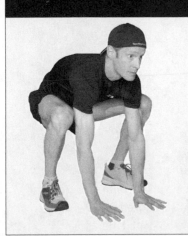

The squatting motion:

It is the most fundamental movement in strength training, and you will see it in various forms in the Hyperstrength workouts. A correct squatting motion is as simple as sitting in an imaginary chair behind you, making sure to keep your weight on your heels and maintaining an erect torso. Bend your knees and slide your hips back until your thighs are almost parallel to the ground, and check your form by ensuring that your knees always stay behind the vertical plane of your toes. (Beginning, out-of-condition, and senior exercisers should start with a half-squat until their exercise form and leg strength improves.) Then simply squat back up.

Triceps Push-up on Knees to Clap: Kneel on the floor and place your hands in a diamond shape on the ground, directly below sternum. Form a straight line from your knees to your shoulders to the top of your head, and keep your feet off the ground. Drop your body down until your arms form a 90-degree angle, then push back up and clap as you balance on your knees.

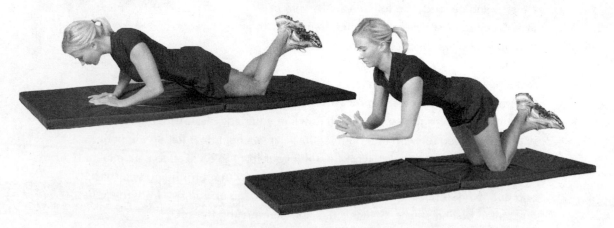

Squat to Dumbbell Overhead Press: Hold the dumbbells at head height with your palms facing out. First squat until your thighs are parallel to the ground (using a chair as a guide), then as you return to a straight-legged position, press the dumbbells overhead.

Alternate Lunge: Stand with your hands on your hips, and then start by taking large steps forward. The lead leg descends until the thigh is almost parallel to the ground, while the back knee almost touches the ground. Make sure the lead knee never goes beyond the perpendicular line formed by the lead toes.

Side-to-Side Squat: First point your right shoulder toward the direction you will travel in. Descend to squatting position and swoop your left hand to the ground, as you side shuffle jump to the right. Repeat for 15 yards, and then switch directions and swoop your right hand to the ground on the way back.

Carioca: Move sideways as quickly as possible by crossing your feet over, first in front and then in back. Once you reach 15 yards, come back facing the same direction.

Straight-Leg Crunch: Lie on your back on a padded surface, with your legs straight and heels on top of the stability ball. With your hands beside your ears, crunch upward by bringing your chest upward and your shoulder blades off the ground.

Oblique Roll-up: Lie on your back on a padded surface and hug the outside of the stability ball with each leg. Stretch your arms overhead to start, then bring the stability ball toward the sky as you roll your body up, one vertebra at a time to 70 degrees.

TREKKER ▲ **Weeks 1 and 2** • **Tuesday/Thursday**

This workout requires access to a running surface. Either use a treadmill (which provides 40% more cushioning than pavement) or, if you are outdoors, use a grassy field (in a park or next to a road) or a dirt trail that preferably has some hilly qualities.

1. Warm-up Jog at 2% incline for 5 minutes (H.E.S. 1)
2. Jog for 5 minutes at 3% incline, then **Dumbbell Squat Kick**, 20 reps (Tuesday, H.E.S. 2; Thursday, H.E.S. 2–3)
3. Walk as fast as you can for 4 minutes at 8% incline, then **Squat Straight Blast Dumbbell Punch**, 30 reps (Tuesday, H.E.S. 2; Thursday, H.E.S. 2–3)
4. Walk as fast as you can for 3 minutes at 10% incline, then 45-second deep breaths (Tuesday, H.E.S. 2; Thursday, H.E.S. 2–3)
5. Walk as fast as you can for 4 minutes at 8% incline, then **Squat Straight Blast Dumbbell Punch**, 30 reps (Tuesday, H.E.S. 2; Thursday, H.E.S. 2–3)
6. Jog for 5 minutes at 3% incline, then **Dumbbell Squat Kick**, 20 reps (Tuesday, H.E.S. 2; Thursday, H.E.S. 2–3)
7. Jump Rope for 5 minutes (30 seconds on/off), H.E.S. 3
8. **Full Sit-up**, 20 reps, **to Child Pose** for 30 seconds; repeat twice

Dumbbell Squat Kick: Assume a boxing stance, with knees slightly bent and feet flat on the floor, one foot in front of the other, and bring the dumbbells to shoulder height, directly beside your cheek. Squat downward, and on the way up kick with your back leg forward (make sure your knee reaches hip height before your foot kicks). Switch to the other side after 20 reps.

Squat Straight Blast Dumbbell Punch: With feet shoulder-width apart and knees slightly bent, hold the dumbbells at chest height with palms facing each other. Do a full squat, then punch with your right hand toward the middle of your body, then immediately follow with left hand. Repeat.

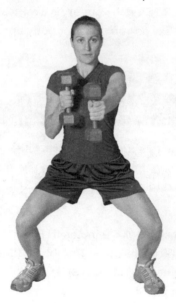

Full Sit-up to Child Pose: Fix your feet under a sofa or bed. With your arms crossed at your chest facing forward, do a full sit-up until your elbows go over your knees. Follow with Child Pose, which begins in table-top position with your palms and knees on the floor shoulder-width apart. Bring your pelvis back to sit between your ankles while your knees spread out and your arms stretch forward, your head remaining in line with your spine.

CLIMBER ▲▲ Weeks 1 and 2 • Monday/Wednesday/Friday

In the drills below, you will perform a set of the first exercise (which is sometimes 2 moves combined) and immediately follow with a set of the second exercise. Take a few reenergizing breaths, then repeat each drill twice more. After 3 sets of each drill, rest for 2 to 3 minutes, and then move to the next one.

1A. **Triceps Skullcrusher to Crunch with Bar Press,** 12 reps
1B. **Medicine Ball Throw to Medicine Ball Slam,** 15 reps

2A. **Dumbbell Holding Push-up with Straight Leg Lift,** 20 reps or 1 minute
2B. **Speed Skater Drill** (holding medicine ball), 20 reps (1 rep is back and forth)

3A. **Barbell Single-Arm Squat Incline Press,** 15 reps
3B. **Rock Climber to Full Jumping Jack,** 12 reps

4A. **Bosu Upside-Down Push-up,** 2 reps, **to Bosu Press,** 10 reps
4B. **Underhand Grip Jump Rings/Bar Pull-up,** 10 reps

IE Drill: Go straight through the 4 drills with little to no rest between them, then repeat twice more (H.E.S. 2–4).

1. **Big Circle Medicine Ball Squat Jump,** 16 reps
2. **Squat Shadowbox Dumbbell Punch with Double Thai Knee Smash,** 15 reps
3. **Quarter-Turn Jump Squat** (moving forward), 30 reps
4. **Knee-high Underneath Claps,** 40 reps

Core: Go straight through the 3 exercises with no rest; repeat twice for 20 reps each.

1. **Stability Ball Crunch** (with Medicine Ball on chest)
2. **Hands Behind Head Stability Ball Sit-up** (bring hands overhead to chest)
3. **Stability Ball Twist** (with Medicine Ball on chest)

Stretch (see pages 58–59)

Triceps Skullcrusher to Crunch with Bar Press: Lie on your back on the floor, holding a loaded straight bar with an overhand grip. With your arms straight and perpendicular to the ground, bend at the elbows and let the bar descend until it almost reaches your forehead, and press back up. Then lower the bar down to your sternum as you raise your chest off the floor, as if performing a crunch, and push the bar straight back up.

Medicine Ball Throw to Medicine Ball Slam: Stand up and hold the medicine ball underneath with both hands. Throw the ball vertically up with as much power as possible. Catch it with both hands in a shot-put position, then bring it quickly overhead and slam it vertically onto the ground. Catch the ball underhanded at waist level and repeat.

Dumbbell Holding Push-up with Straight Leg Lift: Get into push-up position while gripping dumbbells. Do a full push-up, then lift one leg (from the hip joint, keeping your leg straight) as high as possible. Do another push-up, then lift the opposite leg.

Speed Skater Drill: Stretch a jump rope out on the ground. Hold the medicine ball at your chest and get into crouch position with your back curved, like a speed skater. Jump over the rope with your left leg pushing off the floor and land on your right leg, remaining in crouched position, then immediately push your right leg off the floor back over the jump rope to land back on your left leg. Continue until done with your reps.

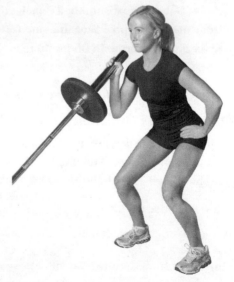

Barbell Single-Arm Squat Incline Press: Load one end of the barbell and place the other end where the floor meets a wall so it doesn't move. Face where the bar is braced and hold the loaded end with one arm at shoulder height. Do a full squat, and then press overhead. Switch sides after completing the set.

Rock Climber to Full Jumping Jack: Get into push-up position. Keeping your upper body fixed, bring your right knee to your chest, then straight again; left knee to chest and straight again; right foot straight out to 3 o'clock and back again; left foot straight out to 9 o'clock and back again. Do this in a staccato, bouncy rhythm. Then jump both feet to under your chest and stand up. Do a jumping jack, then repeat.

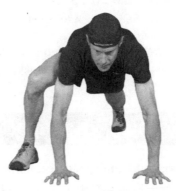

Bosu Upside-Down Push-up to Bosu Press: Turn the Bosu upside down and grip the sides at 9 and 3 o'clock. Do two push-ups, and then jump your feet to under your chest. Bring the Bosu to shoulder level and press it overhead.

Underhand Grip Jump Rings/Bar Pull-up: Squat jump to rings or a pull-up bar and grab with a reverse grip. Do a full pull-up.

Big Circle Medicine Ball Squat Jump: Stand up and hold the medicine ball at navel level. Squat down, then jump up while moving the medicine ball in a big circle clockwise. Repeat 8 times. Then switch and go counterclockwise. Repeat 8 times.

Squat Shadowbox Dumbbell Punch with Double Thai Knee Smash: With a dumbbell in each hand at shoulder height, assume a boxing stance with one leg forward and the other leg back, knees slightly bent, feet flat on the floor. Squat and follow with lead dumbbell hand jab, squat and follow with rear hand, cross (toward the center in front of you, but without hyperextending your elbows). Next, squat and draw your right knee into the center and immediately follow with a squat and left knee into the center, with dumbbells beside cheeks.

Quarter-Turn Jump Squat: Squat and jump forward, turning a quarter turn each jump.

Knee-high Underneath Claps: Run forward, bringing your knees to your chest and clapping your hands underneath each stride.

Stability Ball Crunch with Medicine Ball: With the medicine ball at your chest and your glutes/hips on the stability ball, execute a full crunch.

Hands Behind Head Stability Ball Sit-up: With your hands overhead and your glutes/hips on the stability ball, crunch up to 80 degrees.

Stability Ball Twist with Medicine Ball: Sit on the stability ball and hold the medicine ball with your arms extended in front. Twist all the way to one side and then to the opposite side.

CLIMBER ▲▲ Weeks 1 and 2 • Tuesday/Thursday

This workout requires access to a running surface. Either use a treadmill (which provides 40% more cushioning than pavement) or, if you are outdoors, use a grassy field (in a park or next to a road) or a dirt trail that ideally has some hilly qualities.

1. Warm-up Jog at 2% incline for 5 minutes (H.E.S. 1)
2. Jog for 4 minutes at 3% incline, then **Medicine Ball Wide-Stance Squat and Jump with Medicine Ball,** 20 slow reps and then 20 fast reps (H.E.S. 2–3)
3. Run for 4 minutes at 4% incline, then **Medicine Ball Alternate Leg Lunge and Shoulder Press,** 20 reps (H.E.S. 2–3)
4. Run for 4 minutes at 5% incline, then **Squat Jump with Medicine Ball Overhead,** 30 reps (H.E.S. 2–3)
5. Run for 4 minutes at 5% incline, then **Squat Jump with Medicine Ball Overhead,** 30 reps (H.E.S. 2–3)
6. Run for 4 minutes at 4% incline, then **Medicine Ball Alternate Leg Lunge and Shoulder Press,** 20 reps (H.E.S. 2–3)
7. Jog for 4 minutes at 3% incline, then **Medicine Ball Wide-Stance Squat and Jump with Medicine Ball,** 20 slow reps and then 10 fast reps (H.E.S. 2–3)
8. Jump Rope with 1-pound rope for 5–10 minutes (30 seconds on/off) (H.E.S. 2–3)
9. **Moth to Cocoon** for 20 reps **to Child Pose** for 30 seconds; repeat twice

Stretch (see pages 58–59)

Medicine Ball Wide-Stance Squat and Jump with Medicine Ball: Assume a wide stance and hold the medicine ball between your legs, with your arms straight down. With your back straight and heels on the ground, squat down until the ball touches the ground. Explode up and jump, bringing the ball to your chest as quickly as possible.

Medicine Ball Alternate Leg Lunge and Shoulder Press: Hold the medicine ball to your chest and lunge forward, then press the medicine ball overhead while in lunge position. Return to starting position and repeat on the opposite side.

Squat Jump with Medicine Ball Overhead: Hold the medicine ball directly overhead with straight arms and keep it there throughout exercise. Squat down, then jump up.

Moth to Cocoon, to Child Pose: Hold a light dumbbell in each hand. Lie on your back on the floor, with your legs and arms spread out and with your hands and feet off the ground. Execute a crunch, bringing your knees to your chest and the dumbbells to your feet. Follow with Child Pose, which begins in table-top position on hands and knees. Bring your pelvis back to sit between your ankles while your knees spread out and your arms stretch forward, with your head remaining in line with your spine.

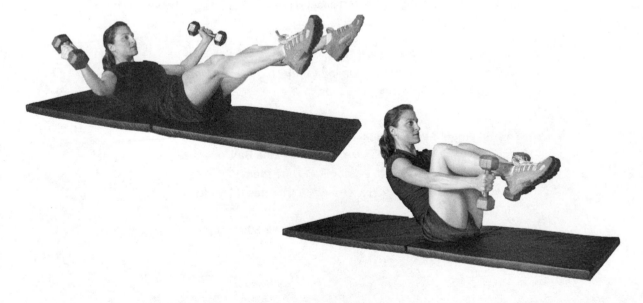

In the 3 intense drills that follow, you will perform a set of the first exercise (which is sometimes 2 moves combined), immediately followed by a set of the second exercise, and then a third exercise. Take a few breaths, then repeat each drill twice more. After the 3 sets of each drill, rest for 2 to 3 minutes (or the time it takes to organize equipment for the next drill) before moving to the next one.

1A. Bosu Push-up with 3-Point Foot Push-off, 15 reps or 1 minute
1B. Angled Squat to 45-Degree Cable Bicep Curl and Jump, 12 reps
1C. Handstand Push-up with One Foot in a Cable Strap, 15 reps or 1 minute

2A. Decline Straps Push-up with 3-Point Stance on Step, 16 reps
2B. Ab Wheel Single, Then Double, 10 reps of each
2C. Squat Jump Touching Floor to Spread Eagle, Then Squat Jump to Daffy, 30 reps

3A. Cable Pullover on Stability Ball, 12 reps
3B. Ski Mogul Master to Fingertip Pull-ups, 7 reps
3C. Push-up to One-Arm Rows and Stand, 8 reps

IE Drill: Go straight through the 2 drills with little to no rest between them, then repeat 3 times more (4 total). Take 30 seconds of deep breaths between each set (H.E.S. 2–4).

1. **Forward to Jump Backward Transition Run** for 30 yards to **Spiderman/Spiderwoman Leaping Climb,** 10 reps
2. **Pop-up to Step Side Jump,** 20 reps

Core: Lying Figure Eight with Medicine Ball, 50 reps

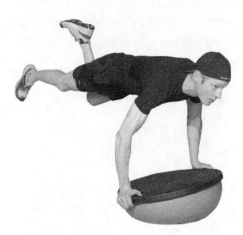

Bosu Push-up with 3-Point Foot Push-off: Assume push-up position with your hands on an upside-down Bosu. Raise one leg off the ground and execute a push-up. Switch feet in mid-air during each push-up.

Angled Squat to 45-Degree Cable Bicep Curl and Jump: Holding two cables, stand with your feet angled out in plié position. Facing straight ahead, do a squat, then a weighted bicep curl. (Weight will vary depending on the individual.) Hold the bicep curl flex for 2 seconds, then jump from plié position to a standard squat position. Repeat the sequence in standard squat position, and shift back and forth to plié position.

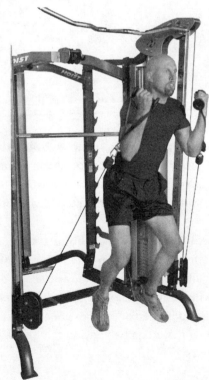

Handstand Push-up with One Foot in Cable Strap: Put one foot into a cable strap, so your body is nearly straight from your head near the floor to your foot in the strap. With your hands shoulder-width apart, do a handstand push-up.

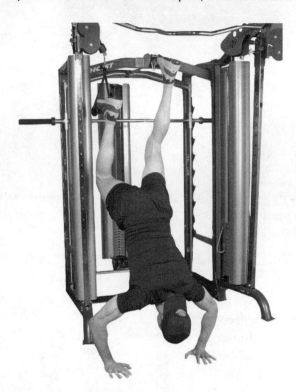

Decline Straps Push-up with 3-Point Stance on Step: With the step and risers higher than the straps (or rings), assume push-up position with your feet on the step while your hands are grasping the strap handles. Complete a decline push-up with one foot off the step. Switch feet after 8 reps.

Ab Wheel Single, Then Double: Use an ab wheel (a compact piece of equipment with one or two wheels in the middle and two handles on either side) or a stability ball (with your hands clasped on top of the ball) and begin on your knees, with your butt directly above your knees and your arms straight. Roll out until your body is straight from your knees to your hands. Return to starting position, and then go halfway and return to starting position. Repeat the sequence.

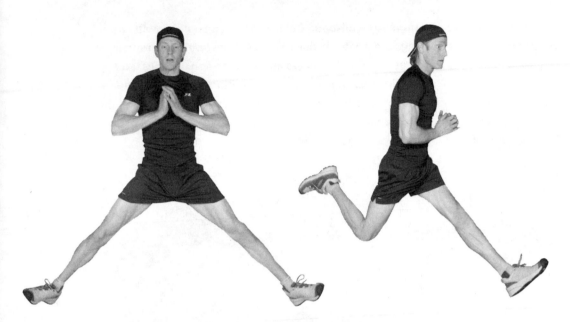

Squat Jump Touching Floor to Spread Eagle, Then Squat Jump to Daffy:
Go down into a squat, and touch your palms to the floor, then jump up and do a
spread eagle with your legs. Squat jump again with your palms touching the
floor, and this time do a daffy—bring one leg in front and the other in back.
During each jump, bring your arms from beside your hips to in front of your
chest. Repeat the sequence, switching legs with each daffy.

**Cable Pull-over on
Stability Ball:**
Grasp onto both
cable handles
attached to the cable
machine at about
mid-height. Sit on
the ball in the middle
and slightly in front
of the cable machine,
then roll down so your head
is closest to the machine and
your knees are farthest away. With the ball firmly
between your shoulder blades, bring both cable handles from behind your
head to the front of your body without bending your arms.

Ski Mogul Master to Fingertip Pull-ups: Get into push-up position, with your feet together. Move your legs quickly from side to side 4 times, with legs remaining together, then jump your legs to spread-eagle position off the floor 4 times, and then do quick jumps by bringing your heels to touch your glutes 4 times. Next, jump your feet to under your chest and stand up. Semi-squat and jump to grab the pull-up bar with your palms facing in; release your grip to only your fingertips holding your weight, and do 4 pull-ups. Repeat the whole sequence.

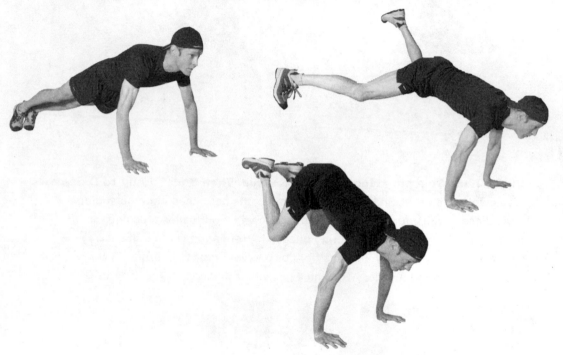

Push-up to One-Arm Rows and Stand: With a dumbbell in each hand, get into push-up position. Do a push-up, then, in extended-arm position, do a one-arm row, bringing your elbow straight back toward the ceiling. Do another push-up, then do a one-arm row with the opposite arm. Do a third push-up, then swing your feet to under your chest and stand up. Repeat the sequence.

Forward to Jump Backward Transition Run to Spiderman/Spiderwoman Leaping Climb: Use a basketball court if possible. Run halfway down backward (bringing your heels to almost touching your glutes), then jump in the air off one foot while turning 180 degrees. Then run toward a wall and leap into it with one foot extended, and attempt to climb up it. Repeat the sequence, alternating the leading leg for the Spiderman/Spiderwoman climb.

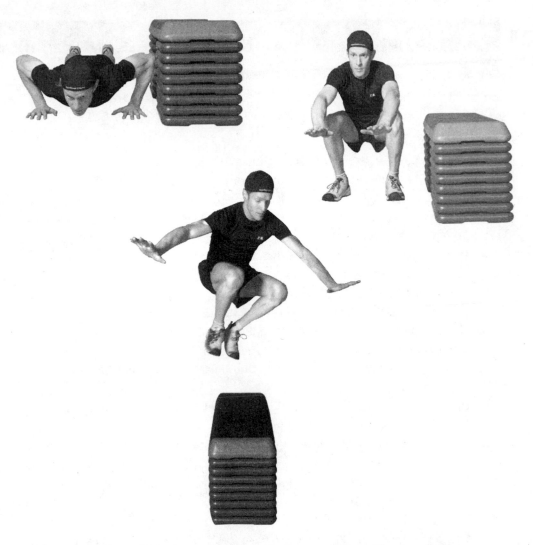

Pop-up to Step Side Jump: Get into push-up position with your chest touching the floor and a step with at least six risers on one side of you. Pop up quickly, jumping your feet to under your chest and arms straight out in front, stand up, then jump sideways over the step. On the opposite side, return to push-up position, pop up, and jump sideways over the step again. Repeat the sequence back and forth.

Lying Figure Eight with Medicine Ball: Lie on your back on the ground, with your legs off the floor. Take the medicine ball and do a figure eight between and around your legs, keeping your feet off the floor.

SHERPA ▲▲▲ Weeks 1 and 2 • Tuesday/Thursday

This workout requires access to a running surface. Either use a treadmill (which provides 40% more cushioning than pavement) or, if you are outdoors, use a grassy field (in a park or next to a road) or a dirt trail that ideally has some hilly qualities.

1. Warm-up Jog at 3% incline for 5 minutes (H.E.S. 1)
2. Run for 5 minutes at 3% incline, then **Decline Stability Ball Core Push-up,** 10 reps (H.E.S. 2–3)
3. Run for 5 minutes at 5% incline, then **Dumbbell One-Leg Squat Big Circle,** 10 reps each side (H.E.S. 2–3)
4. Run for 5 minutes at 7% incline, then **Dumbbell Climb,** 50 reps (both arms up = 1 rep) (H.E.S. 2–3)
5. Run for 5 minutes at 9% incline, then **Jump Split Squat with Dumbbell Shoulder Rotation,** 30 reps (in/out = 1 rep) (H.E.S. 2–3)
6. Run for 5 minutes at 9% incline, then **Jump Split Squat with Dumbbell Shoulder Rotation,** 30 reps (in/out = 1 rep) (H.E.S. 2–3)
7. Run for 5 minutes at 7% incline, then **Dumbbell Climb,** 50 reps (both arms up = 1 rep) (H.E.S. 2–3)
8. Run for 5 minutes at 5% incline, then **Dumbbell One-Leg Squat Big Circle,** 10 reps each side (H.E.S. 2–3)
9. Jog for 5 minutes at 3% incline, then **Decline Stability Ball Core Push-up,** 10 reps (H.E.S. 2–3)
10. Jump Rope with 2-pound rope for 2 songs (quick rests only when completely necessary) (H.E.S. 2–4)
11. **Bosu Squat to One-Leg Hold,** 10 reps, each leg
12. **Climb the Rope,** 2 of 30 reps; **Child Pose** for 30 seconds after each set

Stretch (see pages 58–59)

Decline Stability Ball Core Push-up: With your hands in push-up position and your toes on top of the stability ball, do a push-up and then bring your knees to your chest while rolling the ball toward you. Hold this position for 2 seconds. Then roll ball back out. Repeat the sequence.

Dumbbell One-Leg Squat Big Circle: Hold a dumbbell with both hands, palms facing each other, and stand on your right leg. Perform a one-legged squat, bringing the dumbbell close to your right foot. Come up from the squat and slowly swing the dumbbell clockwise and back down into a one-legged squat. At that point, hop to your left leg and repeat the sequence.

Dumbbell Climb: Hold a dumbbell in each hand. Jog in place so your knees go up high, and raise one dumbbell at a time from shoulder height to overhead with your palms facing the knee that is up, with the opposite arm of the working leg lifting up.

Jump Split Squat with Dumbbell Shoulder Rotation: Begin with a light dumbbell in each hand and one foot in front of your body and the other behind. Keep your elbows anchored to your sides throughout the movement. Begin with the dumbbells faced vertically out to the side, then do a split squat (sinking your pelvis straight down to the ground). Jump and switch feet in midair while rotating the dumbbells inward toward the middle of your body, keeping them vertical. Repeat the sequence.

Bosu Squat to One-Leg Hold: With both feet on the Bosu and arms outstretched overhead, do a squat and touch your toes (without bending your torso forward too much). Watch your fingertips as you bring your hands from your toes to straight above your head, and then hold that pose and stand on one leg for 5 seconds.

Climb the Rope to Child Pose: Lie on your back, with your legs crossed, and your arms stretched above your head. Do 3 overhand grabs at an imaginary fixed rope in front of you, while crunching forward, each grab higher than the next, holding 1 second for each one. Follow with Child Pose, which begins in table-top position, hands and knees on the floor. Bring your pelvis back to sit between your ankles while your knees spread out and your arms stretch forward, with your head remaining in line with your spine.

SHERPA ▲▲▲ **Weeks 1 and 2 · Saturday**

Choose a Recovery workout provided for you in Appendix D, a recovery workout of your own creation, or a sport-specific activity you enjoy, such as basketball, tennis, rock climbing, and the like.

Chapter 4

FINDING YOUR INNER STRENGTH

Weeks 3 and 4

Iɴ ʟᴀᴛᴇ Dᴇᴄᴇᴍʙᴇʀ 2002, I ɢᴜɪᴅᴇᴅ ᴀ client up Aconcagua, the highest peak in South America (as well as the western and southern hemispheres). Getting to the summit wasn't too strenuous, and as I descended to base camp, I couldn't shake the feeling that this mountain had more to offer. For me, mountains provide answers to life's questions, which really are, in fact, my own questions I need to ask myself. When I climb my mind opens wide, and I get in touch with my better, wiser self. Solutions to my problems come naturally, and a peace descends on my restless mind.

There may be a place or an activity that strikes your soul similarly, or perhaps it's the interaction of the two—like cycling through a particularly pastoral bit of countryside or sailing in a body of water when conditions are perfect—which allows you to be truly yourself, and calm and strong at the same time. You'll find that an especially great workout may produce the same result; after doing it for a while you truly will find it hard to imagine why you ever did things any other way.

By the time I settled myself into base camp that night I decided to try a "speed ascent," in which I'd attempt to summit Aconcagua as fast as possible, and then return to base camp the same day. Out of curiosity, as well as to gauge my progress, I looked up the American record for the speed ascent. Up until that point, I hadn't tried to break any mountaineering records, and instead was more interested to see how well my Hyperstrength routines had prepared me for the ordeal at hand. But this time I wanted to test my limits and find out what I had on the inside.

After two days of rest, I rose just after dawn and fueled myself with a huge breakfast. Two hours later, at 8 a.m., I began to speed walk/run from the base of the mountain. I was in a zone, and large blocks of time went by in what seemed like minutes. Just above Nido de Condores at 18,600 feet, I slowed to eat an all-natural energy cookie and noticed my time was only an hour and a half—I was ahead of my projected schedule! Suddenly I realized I had a shot at the record. Any feelings of fatigue disappeared as my confidence level soared, and I continued upward into the rising sun.

I kept pushing it, perhaps harder than I ever had in my entire life. I continued to make great progress by hurdling rocks and keeping my body moving upward. Only an hour from the summit, however, my body started to shut down from the lack of oxygen in my blood and spent muscles. I was desperately exhausted, and for the first time I thought of quitting. As it is on the mountain, which loves to test you in so many primal ways, the weather didn't help matters—it was brutally cold, and the wind was picking up.

But, in spite of the clear message my body was sending me—to turn around immediately—I relied on my **"hy-ki,"** or inner energy, and continued moving toward my goal. Over the eighteen years of my martial arts training and instruction, hy-ki is probably the most important concept that I learned to master. All of us possess hy-ki, but most of us don't know how to access it, or use it to our advantage. But when we can access it, the results are incredible. Hy-ki is not a magic pill, but an energy source that resides deep within you and can only be summoned by specific meditation drills.

My mind and body were screaming, "Give up!" But with my hy-ki, I believed that I could get to the top, and without danger. Rather than continuing to dwell on the pain, I took pride in the fact that my body could handle the test because I had trained for exactly this.

Soon I got to the summit, 22,841 feet above sea level, grateful but exhausted, then descended down the mountain to base camp. I arrived knowing that I had set a new American record. I also knew that it wouldn't have been possible without my hy-ki in my back pocket.

Hy-Ki Helps the Dream

As I've said, I hope this book will inspire you to reach your goals—and not just the cosmetic physical goals, which will simply happen along your Hyperfitness journey. Whether or not you were active before beginning this program, your Inner Everest goal is to make you extra-active in both your fitness life as well as in your pursuit of larger goals.

So I'm going to push you, as you may have already seen in those first two weeks of Hyperstrength. Whether you went with the Trekker, Climber, or Sherpa level, you probably found yourself more physically challenged than you can remember. I hope you were able to complete every workout, and grew to love the exercises—even though they were no doubt challenging!

But at some point, if not already, I know you will struggle. I'm not going to sit here and lie to you. It's part of life—we are human and so we feel a natural resistance to many challenges, no matter how mentally and physically fit we are. That's where your hy-ki can help give you the boost you need.

At this point in the Hyperfitness program, I hope you feel you are on the verge of changing your life for the better. You've demonstrated the mental fortitude and physical readiness to begin this journey, and now is the time to **assess your inner strength.** Ask yourself the following questions:

- When exerting yourself in a significant way, do you consider it painful or exhilarating? Why?
- Do you think of how hard exercising is while you're training?
- Do you breathe from your diaphragm, or does your chest rise when you're breathing?

- If someone makes a negative comment about you or the work you've done on a particular project, does it bother you for the remainder of the day or for a week?

- Do you spend any time by yourself and in silent meditation?

You are about to face the third and fourth weeks of Hyperstrength training, which bring a new series of exercises and IE Drills. Your body will be asked to do more, and the exercises again will be unfamiliar at first. With such challenges for your mind and body, I want you to bring out your inner hy-ki in order to conquer both—and at the same time, I expect you to keep building toward your short-term goal (at the end of the twelve-week program), and your longer-term Inner Everest goal. Learning how to extract this energy and properly channel it will bring you closer to all of your goals, or simply allow you to survive the rough patches. Can you imagine being able to recharge your mental and physical strength at any time? That's what your hy-ki will do for you.

If you came to this program in a "failed" state—such as from a failed exercise regimen, a failed diet, a failed relationship, or a failed job—you may, consciously or unconsciously, find a way to fail at this, too. That may sound

Exercise Performance

BODY CHECK

It's only the third week, but you should already be experiencing an enhanced level of performance—in your workouts, any sporting activities, at your job, and even at home. You're expending a lot of energy in your workouts in order to generate more energy outside of them.

If, however, you don't feel that daily surge of energy when the alarm clock rings, the first minute of the workout, or when you make your first business call of the day, ask yourself the following questions: Have you chosen the right workout level for you? Or do you need to find that inner strength to carry you through the energy low points? It's not too late to downshift to a lower Hyperstrength level, or even to start the program over at the Trekker level. I want you to get the maximum benefit from this program, so you should experience it fully from day one. If that was *not* the case in weeks one and two, then remain on track for weeks three and four, right now. Follow me in getting that hy-ki working.

harsh, but the truth is the only way to a better mind, a better body, and, finally, a better life.

In my first session with prospective clients, I discuss what they consider their "faults"—the junk food obsession, the tendency to blow off exercise commitments, succumbing to the stress at work. It almost always becomes apparent that they are afraid to throw these "crutches" away, like having a crutch to help them walk, even though they're not only unnecessary but impeding them from reaching their goals. While these people can now at least admit that they have such faults, and even know to deal with them in some cases, they have yet to realize that these faults can be erased.

To make sure the past does *not* repeat itself, it's important to adopt a **winning attitude**. Don't confuse this with the "win or else!" philosophy of many maniacal coaches and others. Rather, assume responsibility for your attitude and subsequent actions. Never, under any circumstances, think that you're going to lose at something. Chances are, if you lost a job, had a relationship fall apart, didn't stay with an exercise routine, or performed poorly in a sporting event, mentally, you may have not tried hard enough; losing is when you fail at something and do not learn from it, do not gain or seek knowledge from the mistakes, and do nothing to correct the behavior. But if you learn from such experiences, vow not to make the same mistakes, and continue to give a winning level of effort and attitude, you will never fail, not really.

Up on Aconcagua, I took mental notes of what got me to that exhaustion point, then I re-created that state as often as physically possible in my workouts. I learned to never focus on the pain, for that would only sap my energy; instead, I focused on how exhilarated and invincible challenging exercises could make me feel, plus how they would help enable me to tackle the world's biggest peaks.

The preparation paid off, because I endured extreme pain above 25,000 feet on both Shishapangma and Everest, yet I was able to continue on up the peaks. The aches and pains in my body gave way to my overriding spirit, my hy-ki, which drove me toward the summit somewhere in the clouds above.

At this point, my Hyperstrength workouts are most likely pushing you hard. Eventually, however, you have got to push yourself. To reach your biggest goals in life, it takes Herculean effort—so summon all that you possess within, and finally find what you are capable of.

Hypermind Meditation

Meditation is one of the best techniques for learning to both uncover your hy-ki and unclutter your mind. You have thousands of thoughts every day, and many don't necessarily serve you very well. Daily meditation, for ten to twenty minutes, can put you in a relaxed, focused, and positive state. Common afflictions like stress, anxiety, depression, and headaches—all of which can wreak havoc on your Hyperstrength or Hyperfare routines—are greatly relieved by meditation.

What are the best times to meditate? I recommend either soon after waking up (first go to the bathroom and then take a drink of water), within 30 minutes of eating a meal, the late afternoon, or just before bedtime. Ideally it's a time when you already feel some peace, rather than a tense encounter for example.

Find a very quiet place where you will not be interrupted. Let others know that you are not to be disturbed for the next ten to twenty minutes. Sit in a comfortable chair or lie down on a bed, perhaps with some soothing music playing at a low volume. Close your eyes, and only concentrate on breathing, in and out, feeling your diaphragm rise, not your chest. Have your core fill fully with air, then exhale out through your nose and mouth. Be in the moment, as calm and relaxed as you can be. Let meditation help you focus on the application of breathing for energy. Learn to breathe deeply every day—and it will provide you with an enormous amount of mental and physical strength.

After you become used to the breathing, put into practice one of these three Hypermind meditation sessions. You're welcome to rely on only one of them for your daily meditations, or continually rotate them.

1. **Positive meditation:** Continue to focus on your breathing, and accept that various thoughts will enter your mind. Rather than beginning to analyze

them and allowing them to rouse you out of your meditative state, focus only on the positive emotions and thoughts, while the negative ones slip harmlessly away.

2. **Mantra meditation:** Once again, get yourself in a relaxed state of body and mind. Focus on one sentence, phrase, or word that defines what you stand for. Repeat, over and over again, slowly, focusing on your breathing and the words. Some examples: "I will accomplish my goal." "Do not quit." "Embrace life's energy."

3. **Prayer meditation:** Read a passage from a religious text that you have faith in. Continue to read until you come across a particular verse that strikes you deeply. Say it over and over again, contemplating the words and what they mean to you.

From Martial Arts to Hy-Ki

Ever since I was a boy, I loved watching kung fu on Saturday mornings. I begged my mother to let me take martial art classes, but she preferred to bring me to soccer and basketball practices, museums, and the theater. As I grew older, I knew I needed to channel my energy and confusion as a teenager into something more constructive, and felt martial arts could hold the answers to some of life's questions I had. I got my chance when I entered college and began to study martial arts with master instructor George Craft. His dojo (martial arts gym) became my refuge, and George soon functioned as a second father to me. He had had more than 4,000 students, and out of all of these, he'd only awarded eight black belts. I invested two hours a day, four days a week, to training with him. In my sixth year, my mental and physical perseverance paid off. George presented me with a black belt.

Becoming a skilled martial artist, however, didn't automatically provide me with hy-ki. I had become disciplined with my skills, fitness level, and tenacity, but my emotions remained raw and unpredictable. It wasn't until further years of training with masters in Jeet Kune Do and the Filipino martial arts that I began to understand and manage the true feelings harbored within me for such

Exercise and the Brain

Exercise can certainly benefit the brain, especially in terms of mood and alertness. Several studies back up this claim. In a 2001 *Journal of Sports Medicine and Physical Fitness* study, eighty young male and female volunteers were tested for mood, and then did aerobic activity for an hour. Of the eighty, fifty-two who were depressed before exercising reported a reduction in anger, fatigue, and tension. They also felt more vigorous after the workout.

A famous study conducted at Duke University involved 150 people, age fifty or older, who had been diagnosed with depression. They were divided into three groups and given either exercise as a treatment for four months, the antidepressant drug Zoloft, or a combination of the two. At the end of the four months, all three groups felt better. But the researchers didn't leave it there. They checked again in six months, and the exercise group had relapsed at significantly lower rates than the Zoloft or combination groups. In fact, the scientists concluded that giving the Zoloft along with the exercise undermined the effects of the exercise, suggesting that the combination group would have benefited from knowing that their depression had been lifted as a result of their own exertions, rather than possibly having been brought about by their medication.

a long time. I had to use my reservoir of power in a more virtuous way, and that coincided with my teaching Hyperfitness classes.

By figuring out how to channel hy-ki in productive ways, I was helping people while I was helping myself. I was using my skills and knowledge to change people's lives. In the Hyperfitness classrooms and up on the mountains, it was the same. My hy-ki would fuel me as well as others, as we all become one with the movements. The anxieties, the news of world conflicts and violence, daily hurdles, and job responsibilities would all fade away during this time. I want to see the same scenario for you in our Hyperstrength workouts together.

Mind over Mountain

Having internal strength—or hy-ki—can literally transform your physical performance. The Tendai "marathon monks" of Japan's sacred Mount Hiei, for example, are an amazing illustration of this phenomenon. Over a seven-year period during their training, these monks test the limits of their endurance far beyond

Mastering Lessons from the Monks

Before my ascent up Everest, I visited the monks living at the Tengboche Monastery in Nepal. The lessons they taught me proved to be invaluable—and just as critical as my Western training. Among the techniques they taught me were how to stay focused, release tension, get completely centered, and remain steadfast in pursuit of my goal.

I had read about the monks of the Tengboche monastery for several years. Tengboche is located in the Khumbu region of Nepal at 12,680 feet, and lies on the way into Everest base camp. There you get your first real view of the highest mountain in the world; there I also got my first glimpse of a monk's life, and I've never forgotten it.

The monks would hold daily prayers, and at times they would let us Westerners and other climbers and trekkers view their holy ceremony. They sat in a meditative state, in a large horseshoe-shaped circle in the center of a big room, with a massive Buddha statue near the back wall. Though it was snowing outside, the room was unheated and so it was bitterly cold. I noticed several other climbers shiver, as did I, but the monks seemed oblivious to the drafts. It was my first lesson that would come in handy in the higher altitudes.

On that day, the monks commenced with chanting. I had never heard or seen Buddhist monks chant before, and was immediately moved by the beautiful sounds, which seemed to speak to my soul. Intermit-

tently cymbals, drums, and long blows from a long tube horn joined the chanting. At first the noise was quite atypical to the human ear, but after a while I found it very soothing and peaceful and, oddly, familiar.

Afterward, I gave a small donation to the monks. I watched Sherpas, who had spent the day carrying trekkers' gear from one village to the next, pay homage to the Buddha and pray. I walked outside, where the snow continued to fall and the evening air was crisp. The tremendous prayer experience I had just witnessed had the effect of making me feel wide awake and totally in touch with my core being, so when I stepped out into the snow, I was at peace.

The next day, I struck out for the next village so I could keep acclimating to progressively higher altitudes. I decided to try linking my breathing to a pace while repeating a chant that matched my trekking stride. I mimicked the monks I had heard the night before, and kept a slow, steady hum that started from the pit of my stomach to the outer edges of my lips. I tried this for what seemed like fifteen minutes.

I stopped by a stupa, which is a Buddhist stone shrine, to get some water and relieve my back from the weight of my rucksack. I looked down at my watch to see that I had been trekking for almost an hour and a half. I sat back and smiled, with the knowledge that these monks yesterday had placed another gift in my hands— a gift that I used to scale the tallest peak in the world.

what had been thought possible. They are expected to run 52 miles every day for a 100-day period—that's two marathons back to back!

Such a feat is staggering. But it's possible because of the inner strength of the monks, rather than modern exercise techniques and nutritional strategies. A Tendai monk's running style during those seven years consists of focusing 100 feet in front of him while moving to a continuous rhythm of chant, and keeping his body, especially his head and shoulders, relaxed. And during the fifth year, each monk participates in an ancient running ritual by sitting and chanting mantras for nine days, without sleep or food.

In case you're wondering, joining a monastery isn't my required next step in your Hyperfitness journey, though I certainly wouldn't be against it. Rather, I simply wanted to share with you some of the wonderful lessons that I've tried to apply to my own life—all of which helped shape and define my own hy-ki, and may do the same for you. The monks' ability to train their minds and harness their inner strength is unparalleled.

One can always learn lessons from the world's greatest athletes in terms of perseverance and high-level training, but few in the fitness field have examined how the life of the monk may hold the greatest secrets of all. The desire to win might not be their main motivation, but they reach their goals because of their high level of discipline and belief in their own bodies to perform.

A few years after Everest, I made a decision to try to break the world ascent record up Kilimanjaro. I only did so because I'd learned to apply some of these monk principles into my training program. I'm not a big fan of running constantly—each session on the treadmill used to feel like hours. But after I started chanting during my runs, minutes turned into seconds and, rather than getting increasingly bored during a session, I'd feel as though I was moving, steadily, toward enlightenment.

Putting Your Hy-Ki to Work(out)

With this newfound source of energy available to you, you are now ready to put it into action! While Hyperstrength weeks three and four will force you to step

Chanting During Your Workout

Some monks I met in Nepal could purportedly run up to fifty miles while staring into the horizon by linking their breathing to a specific pace and repeating a chant that matched their running stride. You're not going to run fifty continuous miles (unless that's your Inner Everest goal!), but the use of chanting can significantly boost the effectiveness of your cardiovascular exercises, and even your professional and personal life. Chanting can increase the amount of oxygen you send to your vital organs and muscles each time you inhale. Chanting can make thirty minutes of daily exercise—or any task that had previously seemed overwhelming and time-consuming—feel completely manageable, for deep rhythmic breathing is fundamental to achieving a relaxed state of mind and body. In fact, these same deep, rhythmic breathing techniques are also employed with great success in various natural childbirth methods, such as the Bradley method, which enables a laboring woman to meditate deeply enough to perceive her contractions not as painful but as the natural sensation of muscles doing their work, as do any muscles of the body during exertion.

While jogging, cycling, or rowing at a reasonable pace, try breathing out through your mouth normally, but now try releasing a low, resonant hum from your lips. Do this in rhythm with your breathing, and try to maintain it for fifteen to thirty minutes. With each breath, go deep and try to fully fill your diaphragm. Focus on nothing else but a mark in front of you, and focus your attention on the hum and breathing. This chanting will aid your cardiovascular exercise progress, and you will be able to control the state of your heartbeat better. For example, a more relaxed runner can better preserve his or her energy—a tense one ends up wasting a lot of energy—and utilize it when it's really necessary.

Deep breathing helps you find your hy-ki, and you get none of it when you take shallow breaths, which is quite common among exercisers. Subsequent drills in this book ask you to hold your breath so you can realize that you need to really use those lungs to power you. These drills will build up your overall lung strength.

You can also chant when you are not exercising, for deep rhythmic breathing is fundamental to help achieve a relaxed state of mind and body. Try spending ten minutes a day sitting in a comfortable chair with your eyes closed and doing your slow breathing chant. You will be surprised at how relaxed you are after those ten minutes pass.

up your game another notch, your inner strength—from your hy-ki as well as your hunger for your goals—will drive you through any of the more difficult passages.

Weeks three and four represent your next significant hurdle, and I expect you to go to your hy-ki to bring out a greater level of strength and energy. The more successful you are at doing this, the better are your chances for han-

Don't Let Your Workouts Slip

One way to assure that you hardly ever miss a workout is to be sure you save your energy and time for that workout, rather than squandering it elsewhere. You can so easily dissipate your energy into TV, bad food, surfing the net, or you can put all of your zest into your job but have little left for the workout. Or you can bumble through an unproductive, emotionally negative day and feel like "the last thing you want to do" is exercise.

I've got two responses: first, try moving that workout to the first thing in the day (as I discussed in Chapter Three) so nothing that happens during the day can interfere with it. Second, remember you are guaranteed to feel better after a workout—rather than the same, and certainly not worse. Even if the training session was a slog, and you had to rest more than you wanted, you strained and sweated and made your body feel alive again. As we know, there are few guarantees in life, and even fewer examples of activities that always produce a happier, livelier state at activity's end. Remind yourself that by workout's end, your body will feel lighter and your mind will be comforted by the knowledge that you've done something good for you. It's literally a gift that keeps giving to both body and mind—in the intervening hours before your next workout, your metabolism will be raised, your body fat will decrease, your muscles will grow, and your mind will feel at peace and more able to focus on other tasks at hand as well as on the goals ahead.

dling every workout that comes your way throughout this program and in the future.

When I climbed Everest, I couldn't afford to waste any energy. That's how you should approach each day, with a vigilant effort to remain productive and positive with your energy. Rather than anticipating trouble and making mistakes, don't second-guess yourself or make any excuses. Bring together the powerful energies from your hy-ki and your desire to reach your Inner Everest and short-term goals, and let them both carry you through the daily hurdles and ebbs in your energy levels, including during the workouts. In my experience, the majority of amateur exercisers, unlike pro athletic competitors, don't "bonk" (which describes a body that physiologically shuts down during an athletic performance) as a result of a fluid or carbohydrate problem, but because their minds quit on them. Your hy-ki and your goals won't let that happen, as long as they remain in your mind at the most critical times.

Remember, your workouts are critical! Most people don't stick to their work-

Get More with Mantras

I've seen and experienced how mantras can boost tolerance for sustained physical exertion and maintain positive energy, so I create mantras for both my clients and myself and repeat them constantly. They can provide the additional mental strength and energy necessary to achieve your dreams, and they act as an essential tool in your Inner Everest training. If you keep saying the mantra over and over again, your subconscious starts to believe it. Some examples include "Never quit," "I will succeed," and "No pain."

Mantras also can help you to uncap even more hidden energy and strength, which is especially useful during a challenging session. I have recommended using mantras during several drills in the Hyperstrength program. Don't forget that mantras can be even more valuable to utilize during your daily life, so start creating those mantras now!

Dieting Will Only Slow Your Ascent

As you may know from personal experience or from observation, diets are destined for failure. According to the *American Journal of Clinical Nutrition,* 80 percent or more of diets do not last. Some people try their own "diet" and simply take the "I'm not going to eat as much today!" approach. They'll eat a tiny breakfast, or none at all, and by the time lunch or mid-afternoon rolls around, they'll forget their pledge and they will feel miserable.

Other people fall for the diet gurus and weight-loss programs that are good at selling their products (no matter how inferior for your body their products are). They tell you about "how easy it is!" and the "slimming secrets!" and even that "it's healthy!" But they're lying, because all they're doing is reducing your overall calorie intake, whether it's by reducing carbohydrates, fat, and sweets, or by upping protein. Meanwhile, any energy you might have had for your workouts dissipates with every dieting day.

There aren't that many "secrets" to good nutrition, unless you count the organic, whole-food, no-processed-food approach as radical. If you eat healthy food all the time, it's almost a challenge to *not* lose fat. That's why the concept of diet does not exist in the Hyperfitness world. Diets don't help you lose weight or give you energy. This program is about exercising like an athlete and eating great natural foods.

Hyperfare: The Importance of Breakfast

Simply put, breakfast is the most important meal of the day. I know, you've heard that line before, so it may be easy to dismiss it. So think of it this way: Breakfast is your hy-ki, in the form of food. It should represent your number-one food source of energy, rather than dinner well after most of your day's work is done.

For centuries, farmers understood this. They knew that they'd be toiling in the fields for hours, sometimes taking them too far away from the homestead to make it back for lunch—so a big breakfast was essential for them to work with energy and enthusiasm. It's not rocket science. You've just gone eight or more hours with nothing in your belly, so you require nourishment.

I wouldn't even need to discuss this basic principle if the habit of skipping breakfast hadn't become so common. People either refuse to take the little bit of time they need to have their first meal of the day, or they mistakenly believe that it will help them become thin. It's the reverse, actually—missing breakfast has an immediate, detrimental effect on your metabolism, which naturally slows down because your body is getting this very bizarre message that food isn't coming anytime soon, "so I better hold on to what I got." What you got are fat stores, and they don't go anywhere when your metabolism winds down. Instead, your metabolism desperately needs that breakfast meal to get moving again.

Another stumbling way to begin the day is eating too small a breakfast—especially after a morning Hyperstrength workout, which ideally you began twenty to thirty minutes after a light snack—again thinking that somehow you're going to lose weight this way. Instead, you're usually setting yourself up for major cravings later in the day, or even that morning. And if you make it through to dinnertime without any major indulgences, you "reward" yourself with a big meal. Of course, the evening meal is the one meal that should

outs because they treat them as something extra in their day, something peripheral to their goals, a bonus, if they have the time. Instead, recognize that the Hyperstrength workouts can make the difference between being healthy and unhealthy, living a great life and a could-have-been life, and, inevitably, between life and death.

Hyperstrength, Phase Two: Weeks 3 and 4

At this point, you're probably realizing how relatively easy your former workouts may have been before Hyperfitness—and how unfulfilling. I'm not some sinister drill sergeant who delights in exposing your lack of fitness; rather, I want to share workouts that will bring something special out of you. Even when have the smallest portion size of your day—you don't need the big calorie infusion because the physical part of your day is done. And your metabolism slows down at night and thus stores fat more readily.

You may be thinking, "Okay, I get it: Eat a big breakfast! So we're talking Denny's Grand Slam, right?" Uh, no. Essentially, like all meals, you need a good mix of nutrients to really set your body up for a great day. Too often we load up on simple carbohydrates—white toast, pancakes, bagels, muffins, and doughnuts are a few examples—that predominately contain sugar and yet leave out adequate amounts of protein and fiber. Even the traditional ritual of having a bowl of cereal doesn't give enough nutrition. Protein and fiber are keys in heightening metabolism because they both take longer to digest than simple carbohydrates, so your body is burning more calories while breaking the foods down.

In addition, many of the simple carb breakfasts, like the bowl of cereal with skim milk, have hardly any fat, so you wind up either having a huge bowl (or a second one) or walking out the door still hungry. Satiety, which is created by consuming appropriate levels of the beneficial kinds of fat, is a huge factor in eating the right proportions of food and staying lean.

You should eat carbohydrates that are more complex—they require more time to digest and are also more filling. It's too easy to rifle through three pieces of white toast, but a single slice of an organic whole-grain, wheat-berry bread will do. Go with multi- or whole-grain cereals and breads that are high in fiber and, ideally, organic as well.

In Appendix A, I give many suggestions for Hyperfare breakfasts, which feature all the nutrients I just discussed. Some you can cook—such as an omelet with feta cheese, portobella mushrooms, and organic tomatoes—others you can eat on the run, like an all-natural peanut butter and banana sandwich on whole-grain bread.

you fall a little short during a particular workout, you're getting a taste of what is possible with your body.

In Phase Two of the Hyperstrength program, you will continue to work on muscular and cardiovascular strength, with all levels completing body-weight and free-weight routines. You will continue to battle muscle soreness (learn to embrace it as proof of your progress), yet start to see gains in overall athleticism and lean muscle. Meanwhile, your body fat level will continue to decrease.

The third week involves brand-new exercises, so make sure you follow the exercise descriptions and photos carefully. By the time the fourth week begins, you'll have most of the moves down pat, and the workouts will go by more easily. Training for all levels in these two weeks is designed to build and condition your most important muscle: your heart.

Learn to Run

Like the Bruce Springsteen song, most of us were born to run. However, a majority of those who take to the streets in their jogging shoes have poor technique and more often than not get injured as a result. Here are some ways to become a better runner, when or if you choose:

1. The first rule is to never make running your only form of exercise. Overrelying on running to burn the calories and keep fit isn't smart, because running is not a complete exercise—many parts of your body are either overtrained or undertrained if you run during most of your exercise time.

2. Choose better terrain than pavement to run on. Stick to soft and, better yet, patchy terrain such as grass, trails, and sand. I run on uneven surfaces to burn more calories and strengthen my tendons around my ankles, knees, and hips—and I like to be outside. If you prefer a smooth surface, pick the treadmill; it's not nearly as exciting as outside, but it will save your legs from the pavement pounding.

3. To run faster and with less pounding, work on a higher turnover rate for your feet. You need your nervous system to be trained to run faster. If you fall below 90 strides per minute, practice shortening your stride. Also, maintain a high center and keep your shoulders, hips, and head aligned.

4. No matter how tense your day has been, make sure you relax while running for better efficiency. Relax your jaw, hands, shoulders, and shoulder blades, and let your arms lightly swing back and forth. Like the monks, make running meditative.

Robert B., Sixty-one, Senior Asset Manager

"A year and a half ago I began a new job working in northern Virginia during the week, commuting to my home in Fort Lauderdale, Florida, on the weekends—a schedule I still keep. After finding an apartment to rent, my first item of personal business was to find a gym and a program that would challenge me. After visits to seven different gyms, I was unable to connect with a program that was remotely appropriate and was very discouraged. Then I checked out a health club in northern Virginia, and specifically the programs taught by Sean Burch.

"Unlike most of his students, I knew nothing of Sean's incredible personal athletic accomplishments. I just happened upon the club and him by blind luck!

What good fortune it was, too! I have never been more motivated by a leader or program than Sean's Hyperfitness program, or as satisfied with the results. Last year, at the age of sixty, I ran in the Marathon des Sables in Morocco, and I was physically and mentally prepared to run it competitively, as a result of Sean's example. I am now sixty-one, and have never been in better shape in my life.

"As one of his students, I know Sean to be one of the most extraordinary, creative, and committed persons I have ever met. I, for one, certainly point with pride to my good fortune in being able to work out with him and his Hyperfitness program."

Lori M., Forty-four, Senior Technical Writer

"In the late 1990s, I began working out in the gym for the first time. I found that working out made me feel better. I could cope with life more effectively. I worked a full-time job and exercised.

"Then I got hit by a car and was seriously injured. I lost not only my body strength, but also a part of my will to go on. I crawled back to the gym in the hopes of finding something that would help me recover. I tried chiropractic, acupuncture, physical therapy, balance therapy, massage. I was not much better.

"I'm at the gym one afternoon. I am walking to the water fountain and I see this six-foot-plus redhead teaching a fitness class. I stared, mesmerized and amazed at his strength and tenacity during the class. He had incredible determination, an indomitable spirit, a stunning focus on the moment at hand, and an aura of something—something I couldn't put my finger on— confidence in himself, inner wisdom, dreams, and desire.

"I spoke with this man with the kind eyes and sinewy body and enormous positive energy and found out his name was Sean Burch, and he would help me. And help me he did. We started out with martial arts training and balance drills. Gradually we worked up to boxing, fitness drills, and one-on-one training in his dojo. We trained hard and my body responded in ways I never thought possible. Sean pushed me to my limits. He made me believe I could do things. He wanted me to get better. He was blunt. He would not put up with excuses. He made me a better person physically.

"But the story doesn't end here. Sean's greatest gift to me was his belief in me. I told him that I couldn't go on training unless I worked through issues that kept coming up from my past. He began training me mentally. He listened to me. He started to make me believe that I could dream. Funny, huh? My dysfunctional family life didn't allow dreams. Sean is a dreamer who takes his dreams and makes them a reality.

"Sean climbs mountains. My mountain to overcome is nonpositive thinking. I am a forty-four-year old woman who struggles, just like most women, with body issues. Sean teaches me that unless *you change your thinking,* you *cannot* change your body. He's right. When Sean talks about Hyperfitness, he means to live your life so that you are excited and hyper about it— excited about your goals, your dreams, and your everyday moments. He teaches you to embrace your life in the here and now. He does not preach Pollyanna thinking; he teaches you that struggle is a part of life and quick fixes never work.

"I am writing this testimonial from the heart. I hope someone, somewhere, who is struggling with issues— whether they are mental or physical or emotional— will read this and know that there is someone who can change you. The only thing Sean asks of you is to commit to change and give 100 percent. Not easy. But if you aren't living your life and reaching your peaks, then what are you really doing with your life? Are you surviving or living?

"Sean brought the color back into my life. For this, I am thankful to my dear friend and guide."

TREKKER ▲ Weeks 3 and 4 • Monday/Wednesday/Friday

Go straight through the 6 drills below, 1 minute each, 3 times, with at least 2 minutes rest between each complete round of exercises. For the dumbbell drills, select a weight that will challenge you for 1 minute. If your muscles exhaust before the minute is reached, rest as needed, then continue until 1 minute is up.

1. **Decline Push-up**
2. **Dumbbell Squat to Dumbbell Biceps Curl**
3. **Incline Bench Triceps Push-up,** 2 reps, **to Full Jumping Jack,** 2 reps; repeat the series for 1 minute
4. **Squat One-Hand Shotput Medicine Ball Straight Up to Self-Catch;** 1 minute each arm
5. **Squat Rear Dumbbell Lateral Raise**
6. **Mountain Climbers,** 30 reps, **to Staggered Hand Push-up,** until 2 minutes are up

IE Drill: Repeat the series for 5 total minutes; take 2 full, deep breaths between each drill (H.E.S. 2–4).

1. **Full Jumping Jack,** 20 reps
2. **Backward Jog,** 3 reps, 25 yards
3. **Straight-up Hop Forward,** 20 reps

Stretch (see pages 58–59)

Decline Push-up: Get into push-up position with the top of your feet resting on a step, chair, or bed. Go onto your knees if needed and continue until the minute is up.

Dumbbell Squat to Dumbbell Biceps Curl: Holding dumbbells in each hand, with hands at your sides, perform a squat with legs shoulder-width apart, then follow with a double-arm biceps curl with dumbbells.

Incline Bench Triceps Push-up to Full Jumping Jack: With your hands forming a triangle on a plyo box or bed in front of you, do 2 triceps push-ups. Follow with 2 jumping jacks, making sure to clap your hands overhead and then behind your lower back on the way down.

Squat One-Hand Shotput Medicine Ball Straight Up to Self-Catch: Hold the medicine ball in one hand like a tray, at your side and over your shoulder. Squat down, then push the medicine ball up explosively on the way up. Catch with both hands, and repeat with the other arm.

Squat Rear Dumbbell Lateral Raise: Hold a dumbbell in each hand, with your palms facing in so the dumbbells touch your glutes. Squat down with legs shoulder-width apart, and as you come up, laterally raise the dumbbells to shoulder height.

Mountain Climbers to Staggered Hand Push-up: Get into push-up position. Keep your upper body fixed, then bring your right knee to your chest and then straighten it again; left knee to chest and then straighten it. Do this in a staccato, bouncy rhythm. Then do staggered hand push-ups, which require pulling one hand toward you about a foot, so that it's closer to your kidneys. Do these on your knees if you need to. Stagger your opposite hand the next time through.

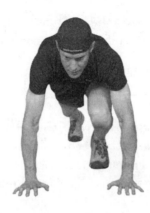

Full Jumping Jack: Execute a full jumping jack, making sure to clap your hands overhead, then behind the lower back on the way down.

Backward Jog: Run backward, trying to hit your glutes with each heel.

Straight-up Hop Forward: Take bunny-rabbit hops (legs and feet together, hopping forward).

TREKKER ▲ **Weeks 3 and 4 · Tuesday/Thursday**

This workout requires access to a running surface or elliptical machine. Either use a treadmill, elliptical machine, or, if you are outdoors, use a grassy field (in a park or next to a road) or a dirt trail that ideally has some hilly qualities.

1. Warm-up Jog at 2% incline or outside for 5 minutes (H.E.S. 1)
2. 2 minutes moderate pace 2% incline, then **Medicine Ball with and without Squat Jumps,** 16 reps; perform the series 3 times total (H.E.S. 2, H.E.S. 3)
3. 2 minutes moderate pace, then **CrossCountry,** 20 reps; perform the series 2 times total (H.E.S. 2)
4. 2 minutes moderate pace, then **Feet Together Side-to-Side, Then Forward and Back over Line,** 30 reps each (forward and back = 1 rep); perform the series 2 times total (H.E.S. 3)
5. 2 minutes moderate pace 2% incline, then **Medicine Ball Toe Taps,** 20 reps; perform series 2 times total (H.E.S. 2, H.E.S. 3)
6. Jump Rope for 4 minutes (30 seconds on/off) (H.E.S. 3)
7. **Straight-Arm Crunch,** 2 sets of 20 reps; **Cobra Pose to Child Pose,** 20 second hold after each set

Stretch (see pages 58–59)

Medicine Ball with and without Squat Jumps: Stand with a medicine ball placed between your feet on the floor. Pick up the medicine ball and squat jump, bringing the medicine ball overhead. Immediately place the medicine ball on the floor and squat jump, bringing only your arms overhead. This equals 1 rep.

Cross-Country: Do scissor kicks in place while making an arm motion like cross-country skiing.

Feet Together Side-to-Side, Then Forward and Back over Line: Make a line on the floor with a jump rope or band. Jump sideways over the line as fast as possible, then forward and backward over the same line.

Medicine Ball Toe Taps: Stand with a medicine ball in front of you on the ground a foot away. Tap the top of the medicine ball with your feet as fast as possible. Switch feet after every tap.

Straight-Arm Crunch: Lie on your back, lock your arms straight out behind your head, interlace your fingers, and cross your legs. Lift your chest and shoulder blades off the floor, while keeping your head and arms in line with your spine.

Cobra Pose to Child Pose: Lie facedown with your feet together and toes pointing behind you. Place your hands flat on the floor and beside your rib cage. Gently push off your hands, lifting your head and chest off the ground and tilting your head back. Feel your chest moving forward as well as upward. For Child Pose, see page 64.

CLIMBER ▲▲ Weeks 3 and 4 · Monday/Wednesday/Friday

In the following 4 drills, you will perform a set of the first exercise (which is sometimes two moves combined) and immediately follow with a set of the second exercise. Take a few breaths before repeating each drill twice more. After the 3 sets of each drill, rest for at least 2 to 3 minutes before moving to the next one.

1A. Cable Lat Pull-down on Bosu, 15x
1B. Chest-to-Floor Medicine Ball Split Squat (left and right side = 1 rep), **to One-Hand Medicine Ball Push-up** (left and right push-up = 1 rep), 8 reps

2A. Dumbbell Squat, to 45-Degree Biceps Curl, to Palms-in Press, 10 reps
2B. Cable Stability Ball Fly, 15 reps

3A. Medicine Ball Triceps Push-up, 2 reps, **to Medicine Ball Squat, to Overhead Press**, 1½ minutes
3B. Scarecrow with Dumbbells and Squat, 1 minute

4A. Pop-up to Full Jumping Jack, 12 reps
4B. Squat Diagonal Dumbbell Press, 12 reps each arm

IE Drill 1: Go straight through the 2 exercises and repeat until 4 minutes are up (H.E.S. 2–4).

1. **Dumbbell Squat Jump on Step,** 10 reps
2. **90-Degree Squat Jump Turns,** 20 reps

IE Drill 2: Go straight through the 3 exercises and repeat until 4 minutes are up. Move forward as you perform these exercises (H.E.S. 2–4).

1. **Frog Jump,** 6 reps
2. **Full Jumping Jack,** 6 reps

3. Tuck Jump to Front, 5 reps

Stretch (see pages 58–59)

Cable Lat Pull-down on Bosu: Grab the cable handles with each hand and kneel on the Bosu placed in the middle of the equipment, without touching your toes to the floor. Bring your elbows toward the sides of your body and squeeze your shoulder blades together. Vary your hand position for each set: 1) palms in, 2) palms out, 3) reverse grip.

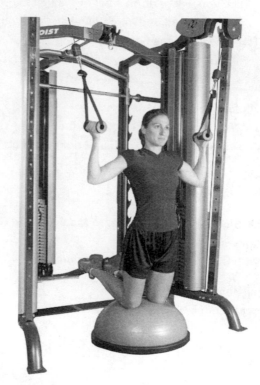

Chest-to-Floor Medicine Ball Split Squat to One-Hand Medicine Ball Push-up: Hold a medicine ball to your chest and assume split squat position (right foot in front and left in back). Squat down and bring the medicine ball from your chest to the floor on your left side. Once the ball reaches the floor, jump up and switch legs, bringing the medicine ball from your chest to the floor on your right side. Next, go down into push-up position, with one hand on the medicine ball and the other hand on the floor, and do push-ups on both sides.

Dumbbell Squat, to 45-Degree Biceps Curl, to Palms-in Press: With dumbbells at your sides, do a squat, dumbbells lightly touching the floor, then follow with a biceps curl as you rise from the squat and, finally, press the dumbbells overhead with your palms facing each other and rise off your heels. Reverse slowly on the downward movement.

Cable Stability Ball Fly: Lie back on the stability ball, firmly positioned between your shoulder blades. With a cable in each hand and straight arms, place the cable handles directly above your rib cage. Bring the cable handles back out to sides until you feel an outer stretch.

Medicine Ball Triceps Push-up, to Medicine Ball Squat, to Overhead Press: Do 2 triceps push-ups on the medicine ball, then jump your feet together. Squat down with the medicine ball at your chest, and then press overhead as you squat up.

Scarecrow with Dumbbells and Squat: Hold a dumbbell in each hand, with both arms bent at 90 degrees (one down arm and the other up, like a scarecrow). Squat and change arm positions at the bottom and during each squat.

Pop-up to Full Jumping Jack: With arms bent in push-up position, chest flat on the ground, and legs straight, pop feet under chest and explode up into a jumping jack, making sure to clap hands overhead and then behind lower back on the way down.

Squat Diagonal Dumbbell Press: Begin in a squat position, with one dumbbell in your right hand placed near the inside of your left foot. Stand up while bringing the weight diagonally across your body to overhead. Switch sides after the set.

Dumbbell Squat Jump on Step: Use at least 4 risers for the step and hold a dumbbell in each hand, palms in and at shoulder height. Facing the step, go into a squat position and jump onto the step. Step back down, and then repeat.

90-Degree Squat Jump Turns: Facing sideways to a step with at least 4 risers, and hands on top of your head, squat jump and turn 90 degrees in the air to land on the step. Step down on the opposite side and repeat.

Frog Jump: With your hands on top of your head, squat down to 90 degrees with your legs and rise, hopping forward, two feet at a time.

Full Jumping Jack: Execute a full jumping jack, making sure to clap hands overhead, then behind lower back on the way down.

Tuck Jump to Front: Jump up, quickly, bringing your knees as close to your chest as you can.

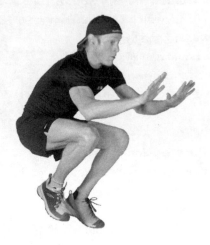

CLIMBER ▲▲ Weeks 3 and 4 • Tuesday/Thursday

This workout requires access to a stationary bike, or you can use a treadmill and perform moderate (H.E.S. 2–3) paced runs in place of the cycle portion in this series of drills.

1. Warm up 5 minutes at moderate pace, 70 rpm (H.E.S. 1)
2. **Side Squat Launch,** over step with risers, 40 reps
3. Low resistance, high cadence turnover on bike, 110 rpm for 2 minutes, slower for 30 seconds; perform the series 4 times total (H.E.S. 3; H.E.S. 2 on recovery)
4. **Flashdance,** move forward for 20 yards. You should make 100 steps total before getting to the other end. Take a 20-second rest in between. Perform the series 2 times total (H.E.S. 2–3)
5. Medium resistance steady cycle one song, then sing the next song out loud while keeping an aerobic cadence (H.E.S. 2–3)
6. High resistance, out-of-saddle steady climb on bike for 2 minutes, and then down in the saddle for 1 minute (same resistance); perform the series 3 times total (H.E.S. 3)
7. **Bounce Squats,** 5 times, **to Jump Squat, to Push-up Position,** to Jump, 15 times (H.E.S. 3)
8. Jump Rope with 1-pound rope for 2 minutes (while jumping, jog in place to feet together side-to-side); perform the series 3 times with minimal rest when needed in between sets (no more than 15–30 seconds); put a photograph of a goal on the wall in front of you while jumping (H.E.S. 3)
9. **Crunch, to Leg Lift, to Side Crunch;** 20 times each; perform the series 2 times, no rest
10. **Downward-Facing Dog Pose to Superman,** 5-second hold in each position; perform the series 4 times

Stretch (see pages 58–59)

Side Squat Launch: Stand sideways to a step with at least 5 risers, with one foot on top. As fast as possible, bring the other foot on top of the platform, then bring the first foot to the opposite side and touch the ground with your hand. Each time a foot and hand touches the ground, squat, leaving one leg on the step. Go back and forth.

Flashdance: Go forward with fast feet, as if the ground were scalding hot.

Bounce Squats, to Jump Squat, to Push-up Position, to Jump: Bounce squats are quick pogolike jumps beginning in a squat position; then do a jump squat from a lower squat position, with your thighs parallel to the ground; then go to push-up position; come up and jump as high as you can.

Crunch, to Leg Lift, to Side Crunch: Lie on your back on a mat with your legs crossed and crunch upward to 45 degrees. Next, bring your legs up and out for your lower abs; last, bring each elbow across your body to touch opposite knees.

Downward-Facing Dog Pose to Superman: Start on your hands and knees with your back flat and head in line with your back. Curl your toes under and straighten your legs, and then push upward with your arms. Lengthen your spine while trying to keep your legs straight and feet flat on the ground. Your weight should be evenly distributed between your hands and feet. To go into the Superman position, start by lying facedown on the floor. Extend your arms so they are parallel to the floor. Then, lift your arms, head, chest, and legs (from the hip joint) off the floor.

SHERPA ▲▲▲ Weeks 3 and 4 · Monday/Wednesday/Friday

In the following 3 intense drills, you will perform a set of the first exercise (which is sometimes two moves combined), immediately followed with a set of the second exercise, and then a third exercise. Take a few deep breaths, then repeat each drill twice more. After the 3 sets of each drill, rest for at least 2 to 3 minutes (or the time it takes to organize equipment for the next drill) before moving to the next one.

1A. **T Push-up, to Twist Push-up, to Shoot Push-up, to Feet Together with Dumbbells** (6 push-ups with various moves = 1 rep), 5 reps

1B. **Towel Pull-up on Stability Ball,** 15 reps

1C. **Iditarod,** 20 reps

2A. **Flapping Bird,** 15 reps

2B. **Aerial Spin over Steps,** 20 reps

2C. **One-Leg Kettlebell/Dumbbell Squat to Overhead Press,** 10 reps on each leg/each arm

3A. **Decline Push-up with Feet in Rings/Straps with Swoop Rolls,** 12 reps

3B. **Punch Mitt Strike** (4 hits = 1 rep), 10 reps

3C. **Decline Bench Barbell from Overhead to Forward Extension Sit-up,** 15–20 reps

IE Drill: Repeat the series for 12 minutes. Take 30-second deep breaths and yell one mantra between each drill. The time allows for 2 series (H.E.S. 3–4).

1. **Alien Run** for 20 yards, **to Full Jumping Jack, to Frog Jump,** to back to start; repeat the series 8 times total

2. **Pop-Up over Step, to Alien Run** for 20 yards, **to Backward Frog Jump,** to back to step; repeat the series 6 times total

Core: Flutter Kicks, 30 reps, to Circles, 10 reps clockwise and 10 reps counterclockwise, to Sit-up, 5 counts on the downward movement, 15 reps; perform the series twice, no breaks (do Monday and Friday only)

Stretch (see pages 58–59)

T Push-up, to Twist Push-up, to Shoot Push-up, to Feet Together with Dumbbells: With a dumbbell in each hand, do a push-up and put all of your weight on one straight arm while the other arm remains straight overhead (forming a T); do another push-up and repeat on the other side. Next, do a push-up and then twist your torso, bringing one dumbbell underneath and across your body as far as possible (palm will be facing up); do another push-up and twist to the other side. Next, do a push-up and bring one dumbbell out straight in front of you, then do another a push-up and repeat on the other side. Then, bring your feet under your chest, and stand up holding the dumbbells.

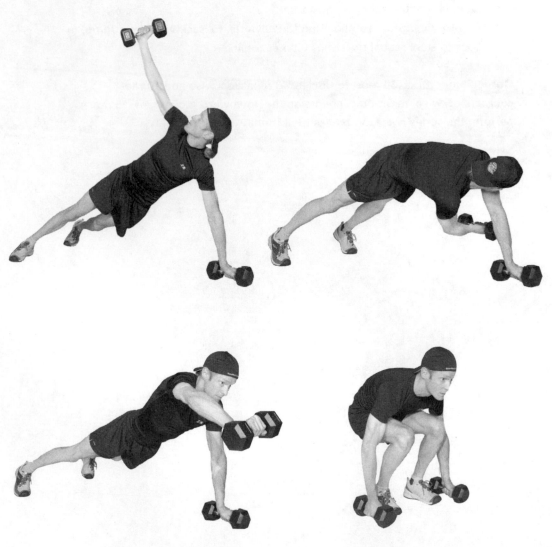

Towel Pull-up on Stability Ball: Drape two towels over a fixed bar/rings/straps to use as handles, while your body is off the floor and both heels are on a stability ball. Drop your glutes down until your arms are straight, then pull your chest up toward the bar/rings/straps.

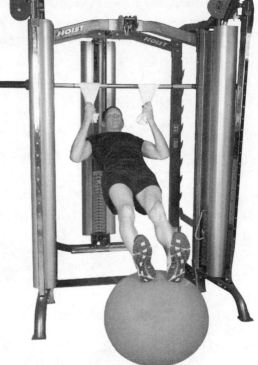

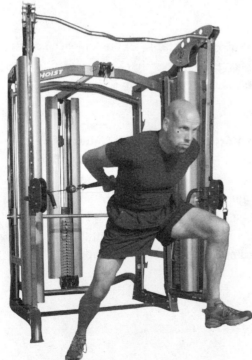

Iditarod: Face away from a cable, with both hands holding the cable handle at hip height behind your back. Jump forward diagonally, pushing off with one leg, then step back and jump to the other side diagonally, pushing off with the other leg.

Flapping Bird: Lie on your back between the cables, with the handles on a low pinhole. Legs are elevated and bent at 90 degrees. Grab the handles and bring in until they meet under your hamstrings while lifting your chest off the floor toward the ceiling.

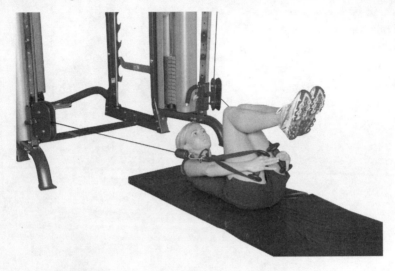

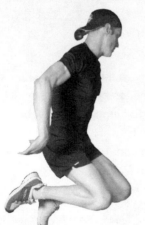

Aerial Spin over Steps: Set up at least 3 steps with at least 8 risers (or other obstacles), do complete 180-degree spin jumps over it and then back again.

One-Leg Kettlebell/Dumbbell Squat to Overhead Press: With one leg on the floor bent at 90 degrees and the other foot off the floor and behind you, hold a kettlebell or dumbbell down at your side and squat down. Touch the floor with the weight, then squat up and press the weight overhead.

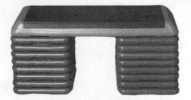

Decline Push-up with Feet in Rings/Straps with Swoop Rolls: Place your feet in rings or straps, and then do push-ups with a swoop at the bottom of each one, shifting your weight from left to right, raising your opposite hand at the top, and then swooping to the opposite side.

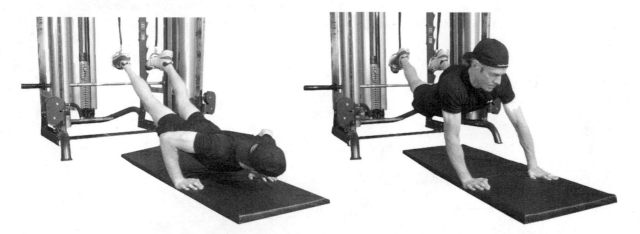

Punch Mitt Strike: Stand arm-length away from the wall, with a heavy medicine ball in your hands. Squat down and then aggressively squat up and push out the medicine ball from chest level into the wall, without it leaving your fingertips. Hit four different points on the wall after each squat.

Decline Bench Barbell from Overhead to Forward Extension Sit-up: Lie down on a decline bench with a barbell overhead. Do a forward extension sit-up and bring the bar all the way to your shins.

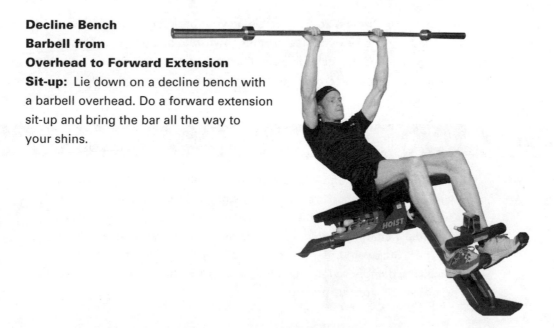

Alien Run, to Full Jumping Jack, to Frog Jump: Run on all fours with your hips staying low. Follow with a jumping jack (making sure to clap hands overhead, then behind your lower back on the way down) and a frog jump: with your hands placed on top of your head and your feet slightly angled out, squat down until your glutes are almost near your ankles and your knees go out in the same angle as your toes; then explode forward, jumping like a frog.

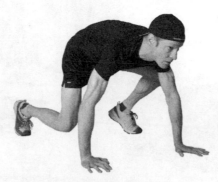

Pop-up over Step, to Alien Run, to Backward Frog Jump: Lie facedown with your head closest to a step with risers. Pop up and jump over the step, then alien run 20 yards down and come back frog jumping backward (with your hands on your head), then jump back over the step.

Flutter Kicks, to Circles, to Sit-up: Lie on your back on a mat with your feet 2 feet off the floor and kick your feet up and down with straight legs. Then put your feet together and do circles in each direction. Last, do full sit-ups with your hands behind your head and one foot over the other.

SHERPA ▲▲▲ Weeks 3 and 4 · Tuesday/Thursday

1. **Frog Jump** forward and back down a basketball court (or 30 yards) 1 time while holding dumbbells at shoulder height, then **Dumbbell Push-up to Overhead Press,** 10 reps, then sprint down and back the basketball court (or 30 yards) 1 time while holding dumbbells; perform the series 5 times total.

   Then, **Stairwell Drill** (if there's no stair access, then high-knee jog in place with dumbbells for 4 minutes); run up 1 flight of stairs while holding dumbbells, 5 times up and down.

Next, get on the treadmill: 15% incline with dumbbells, walking fast for .25 miles, 10% incline without dumbbells, running for .50 miles, 15% incline with dumbbells walking fast for .25 miles

Perform this entire series of drills 2 to 3 rounds, depending on time needed to complete each round (H.E.S. 2–4).

2. Jump Rope with 2-pound rope for 3 minutes

Core: Flutter Kicks 30 reps; Circles, 10 reps clockwise and 10 reps counterclockwise; Sit-up, with 5 counts on the downward movement, 15 reps; perform the series twice without breaks

Stretch (see pages 58–59)

Frog Jump: With your hands on top of your head, squat down to 90 degrees with your legs and rise, hopping forward, two feet at a time.

Dumbbell Push-up to Overhead Press: With a dumbbell in each hand, do a push-up. Next, bring your feet under your chest and stand up, pressing the dumbbells overhead with palms facing out.

Stairwell Drill: Using a stairwell between 2 floors of a building or stairs with at least 25 steps, run up 1 flight of stairs while holding dumbbells, 5 times up and down. If there is no stair access, then high-knee jog in place holding dumbbells for 4 minutes.

SHERPA ▲▲▲ Weeks 3 and 4 • Saturday

Choose one of the Recovery Workouts provided for you in Appendix D, a recovery workout of your own creation, or a sport-specific recovery workout.

Chapter 5

EMBRACE THE UNKNOWN— VANQUISHING FEAR

Weeks 5 and 6

In ANOTHER TRAINING EXPEDITION for Everest, I journeyed within the Arctic Circle to Greenland, which has some of the most compelling (for a mountain climber) virgin peaks in the world. With modest altitudes, unpredictable weather, and little human support, it was perfect preparation for the Himalayas.

Climbing with a British expedition team, I enjoyed getting up several first ascents (peaks that had never been ascended before) in a very controlled, systematic fashion. We accomplished exactly what we had plotted out for ourselves, and everyone was ready to head home—everyone, except for me.

I decided to toast the expedition's success by doing some first ascents with a climbing partner. We headed out into the vast Arctic on the last day feeling overcome with anticipation and nervousness. By early morning, we had succeeded at a few first ascents and were feeling, literally, on top of the world. These climbs, though rewarding, still left something to be desired, and many summits remained unclimbed. I felt these steep peaks tug at my heart, daring me to climb their summits on my own.

Because of Greenland's remoteness, solo ascents are considered taboo. No one was tempted, because it would mean climbing at your own peril and knowing that if you were seriously injured, you'd have an arduous chance of getting out alive.

I decided to head out to climb one more solo first ascent (having completed one earlier in the expedition), and reached the mountain's summit just as the pale gold morning sun was melting into the blue sky above the polar icecap. Heavily fatigued and hungry, I was looking forward to food and my sleeping bag back at camp. Unable to rope myself to any climbing partner, I had been extremely careful throughout the ascent, but during the final descent I began to relax, thinking all I needed to do was follow my tracks back down the mountain. My focus began to drift, influenced by my mental and physical fatigue.

Suddenly, without knowing it until it was too late, I stepped through a snow bridge. My crampons (spikes attached to the bottom of boots) punched through the thin layer of crusty snow, and the ground dropped away like a freight elevator cut from its cables. I plunged up to my armpits into nothingness, and then found myself sinking fast in loose, quick-shifting snow that sucked at my body like quicksand. Instinctively my arms shot out from my sides to fight the pull, and then it dawned on me: I was sinking into a crevasse that seemed intent on swallowing me whole.

My life began exploding before my eyes. It was as if every memory was in slow motion, yet everything else was happening way too fast. This was not how I wanted my first trip to Greenland to end, dying alone in a crevasse—another example of a climber hell-bent on doing it his own way.

With fear nearly overwhelming me, I took a quick breath and remembered the ice ax in my right hand. I summoned all of my mental and physical training to pull myself vertically out of the frozen tunnel. Extending the ax as far as I could reach on the crest, I anchored it into the ice with an overhead chopping motion. Then, little by little, I began to pull myself out of the crevasse.

Once on solid ground, I laid down in the snow, panting for breath. Looking toward the edge of the black void that had nearly devoured me, I realized how close to death I'd possibly come. I knew that fear, awakening my body to its highest level, had forced me to act and had saved my life.

Rather Than Letting It Abuse, *Use* Your Fear

I had never come that close to being on the thin line between life and death before. My mountaineering skills were put to the ultimate test, and they passed, barely, helped by that intrinsic human instinct called fear. Instead of getting crippled by fear and losing my life, fear gave me the energy to extract myself from the abyss.

I believe that the ability to use fear to your advantage rather than your disadvantage is one of the primary reasons why some people succeed and many others struggle—in both dire situations and everyday ones. How can you use fear to your disadvantage? Well, look around: Many people use fear to block progress toward their goals—whether it's committing to an exercise program or to another person, to pursuing a promotion or new business venture, to going on an adventure expedition or a human rights mission, or some other goal.

But I want you to learn how to use fear—those feelings of dread, anxiety, and self-doubt that can flood your mind, often at critical times—to your advantage. Often we think our own personal fears are embarrassing and unique (no wonder they can debilitate us!), though they are usually quite normal and common. So face them, with the knowledge that many people you admire in your life—as well as the history of the human race—have lived with the same fears or very similar ones.

I'm talking about benign fears, like hesitating to talk to someone you're attracted to, and major ones, such as finding out that you've just been diagnosed with a life-threatening illness. In 1996, my best friend, Joseph, got lymphoma, a type of cancer that spread havoc throughout his upper respiratory system. After seemingly defeating the disease, it came back in 1999. This time around, Joseph had to receive chemotherapy ten times as powerful as the first dosages and, if he survived the chemo, faced a bone marrow transplant. He endured the chemo and the bone marrow transplant, emerging at the other end of an absolutely grueling, terrifying year a cancer-free human being. He faced his most morbid fears, twice, and resolved to fight with as much will and strength as he could muster. It was enough, for today he remains a healthy man, with a wonderful wife and three children.

I asked Joseph what the most important lesson was that he learned from his battle with cancer. He smiled, and said, "There are so, so many. Never sweat the small stuff. When I get stressed out at work, or complain about life's problems, all I need to do is close my eyes and imagine myself back in the hospital. I was so scared of the cancer, losing my life, my children not having a father, of many things. There was a day, in the middle of my treatments, when I looked in the mirror in my bathroom: my hair was gone, there were tubes sticking out of my chest and my arms, and I had lost all muscle tone in my body. I looked completely unrecognizable to myself. I knew there was only one goal I had to focus on—defeating cancer—and I did. This also gave me perspective on life. Owning material possessions is nice, but they don't mean as much to me anymore as they once did. I think of that moment in the hospital, and it helps remind me that health, wellness, and family are what matter most. Being fearful is a natural progression. We all feel it, but it's how you react to your fears that matters."

Have you ever noticed that that expression "Face the facts" is inherently negative, as in, "Give up, pal, the odds are stacked against you." Well, after getting cancer a second time, Joseph turned the meaning of that expression on its head, essentially saying, "If I beat it once, I can beat it again." He was right.

The facts or the odds don't always favor our attempts to win the race, get the raise, or get the part—*unless you decide that they do.* Believing that will help you work harder than anyone else you're competing against, because you will know that you belong on top of that podium.

Of course you don't have to be confronted by death or life-changing issues to understand the power of fear, just as you don't have to put yourself in danger in order to conquer your fears. Experiencing fear can be as simple as competing in a road race for the first time, or going into your boss's office and asking for that raise that you rightfully deserve. Fear can be as basic as driving on a high-speed expressway or getting caught in a thunderstorm walking home from the grocery store. Consider Maria T. (see page 129), a thirty-four-year-old elementary school teacher and client of mine, who used to get so nervous before my class that she would literally grow sick to her stomach. She overcame that fear, and now is in the best shape of her life.

Similarly, my desire to climb Mount Everest stayed within me for four long years before I finally decided to conquer my fear of heights, address my mountaineering inexperience, and begin my journey toward the summit. Now, having climbed to several dozen high-altitude summits around the world, I'm *again* making up for lost time.

You may also have had some fears that kept you from enjoying or prospering in different areas of your life, perhaps for many more years than you'd care to recount. Don't look back with regret, as that will do you no good; instead, look back and learn, then decide to face those inner challenges (which is what fear really is) today. Were the goals that you wrote down on your self-discovery journey in Chapter One established right then or have they been with you for many years? Many goals take a while to achieve—like buying a home, starting your own business, or writing a novel—so get started now in overcoming the fears that have kept you from making progress toward these goals. Don't put it off any longer! The more you avoid or postpone facing your fears, the more they will build upon themselves.

A mastery over your fears, along with the hy-ki we accessed in the last chapter, will become critical as your journey to reach your Inner Everest continues.

I Was Once Ruled by My Fears

Growing up, I was terrified to ask a girl out on a date, to speak up in public, and to tell someone I was mad at them; I also had an inescapable feeling that I would never find anyone to love unconditionally. I kept these fears to myself, avoiding them as much as I possibly could.

By the end of my twenties, I'd made headway with some of those fears, yet was still ruled by them in the love department. I'd fallen hard by a couple of close relationships and had become unwilling to devote myself completely to someone.

I can almost laugh about some of those relationships now, but, back then, breakups reconfirmed all my fears about relationships: that I would never find anyone whom I could trust, and certainly never anyone who "got me," as in, understood who I was and really cared. The heartache was so palpable, I felt like

What Fear Has to Do with Why Some People Are Out-of-Shape

Fear is one of the primary reasons that some people aren't healthy. It's behind the horrible low-impact, moderate-exercise trend that took over a couple of decades ago. "Hey, let's make sure we don't get injured and don't challenge our bodies too much. Let's exercise like we're all one step into our graves!" Imagine how well that would work for the cheetah or the wildebeest.

Some people might say Hyperfitness is "too extreme" and "not for your everyday exerciser." That's fear talking! "Extreme" compared to what I see in health clubs and exercise DVDs? "Too hard" for an exerciser who prefers to walk from one easy machine to the next, barely breaking a sweat? Yeah, I hope so! A majority of today's fitness trends are for obese people who want to remain obese, because many people are afraid, and they're unwilling to work harder. I read an article in a fitness magazine the other day that listed "the only five exercises you will ever need." That's the same as saying that all you need to do to stay fit is walk for thirty minutes three times a week, or do an eight-minute abs program. Oh, you've heard that already?

With Hyperfitness, you can burn ten times the number of calories in an hour than the majority of other programs; you can become the athlete that you've always wanted to be, no matter what your age. If you can hang with the Hyperstrength workouts, the rest of each day will seem like a piece of cake. So stop listening to fearmongering about challenging fitness, and find out what your body and mind are really capable of—the possibilities are limitless.

my heart would bleed through my skin. I threw my mind and body into my work and fitness, in order to negate any possible long-lasting, meaningful relationships.

Then, another blow to my already pessimistic view of relationships hit: my parents, after twenty-nine years, were getting divorced. After my father moved out, I moved in to keep my mother company and help her move on. Every night, after our separate workdays, I'd cook up a great, healthy meal for us, and we'd talk about our days, our thoughts, and our troubles for hours. We were always close, but during the year I stayed there we became best friends.

By the time I struck back out on my own, I was almost ready to be in a relationship again. My mother kept telling me that in order to truly experience life I had to be willing to make myself vulnerable again. I wasn't entirely convinced until one day I met a woman named Gabrielle. She was such a positive, vibrant, and intelligent person—and I'd never come across anyone quite like her before. But I remained gun-shy, even pleading with her not to date me. Not only did I feel I was not ready for a relationship but I really was afraid to change.

We casually dated, on and off, for almost a year. We would tell each other our dreams, and she'd always listen with a smile and caring soul. She seemed to understand my mental distress but was not defeated by my gloomy take on long-lasting relationships. Every now and then, she would call to just say hello; many times, we'd simply get together to chat about life and the issues of the day. When I would go inward, she never got perturbed; yet, when I had to spill my guts about something, she'd take the time to listen, without judging, and would offer encouragement and sensible advice.

She constantly gave me positive reinforcement about my dream of climbing Everest, and encouraged me to go on preparatory climbs around the globe. She knew my faults—how could she not—but didn't try to change me; rather, she accepted who I was and, even better, liked what she found.

But despite all our time together, I remained reluctant to immerse myself in another relationship. She seemed to understand that I was still afraid to give myself over to someone entirely.

My expedition to Ecuador served as the turning point. Out in full-blown Mother Nature, after being cooped up in the city and my job and my house for too long, I felt more relaxed than I'd been in a long time. But something, or more like someone, was missing. I couldn't get Gabrielle out of my head, and I realized how much I really loved her.

When I got off the plane, I saw her smiling face and was overjoyed, an emotion that I hadn't felt in so long. I decided on our drive back to my house to let myself go, and begin changing my attitude about relationships and overcome my fear of becoming emotionally entangled again. I became willing to admit that I was wrong about relationships, but right about Gabrielle. She had rescued me from me countless times. I wanted now to be someone she could trust and depend upon, as I had depended on her for so long.

Most people who meet me today, or who have known me only within the past five years, assume that the way I act now is the way I have always been. Nope—the Hyperfitness testimonial starts with me, because I live my life entirely opposite from how I did back then. I made a decision to finally face my fears, knowing my goals would never become reality if I didn't. Today, not all of my fears are gone—and some of them help keep me alert and active—but they don't hamper me like they once did. Now, fear lets me know I'm alive, and I try to always embrace the unknown.

Taking an Unflinching Look at Your Fears

It's easy to brush off reality in your brain, but harder when you have put your anxieties down on paper. I want you to assess your fears and how you respond to and deal with them on a daily basis. There are no right or wrong answers; rather, your answers should help build critical self-awareness and self-knowledge.

In the first series of questions, I would be surprised if you didn't write yes next to at least a few. Seven years ago, I answered yes to all eight questions. Getting in touch with your fears will allow you to ameliorate them, one step at a time.

It is only natural to have fears in your life. However, in the second series of questions, if you answered yes to any of the three, then you may be letting fear control your life and, therefore, your dream goals. No single fear, person, or situation should have that kind of power over you.

The first set of questions demonstrates fear as a constant energy that will always be with you in some shape or form. The second tier of questions is to help you realize that you can deal with fears in two very different ways: either as a motivator or roadblock.

Three Ways to Conquer Fear

Fortunately, there are at least three concrete methods for turning fear into strengths. Too many of us have allowed fear to cripple our attempts to succeed in different ways, so the first method I recommend is to **treat fear as a positive force.** It's really all about perception, as I've learned to value fears and even look forward to them each day. Why? Fear can make you feel alive! Fear can give you energy when you thought you were completely exhausted; fear can push you to

Question	Yes/No	Is this fear manageable? Yes/No
Do you fear illness and/or death?	____	____
Do you fear social situations?	____	____
Are you afraid of embarrassment or failure?	____	____
Do you fear crime/violence/becoming a victim or a biological/chemical attack (terrorism)?	____	____
Do you have any phobias (e.g., are you terrified of heights, driving, being alone)?	____	____
Do you fear getting injured and going to the hospital?	____	____
Are you afraid to speak in public?	____	____
Are you afraid of relationships?	____	____

What are the fears you feel are holding you back? List them here:

1) _____

2) _____

3) _____

4) _____

5) _____

Now place each of your fears in context with the three questions below:

Question	Yes/No
Do you spend at least a quarter of your day thinking about your fears?	____
Do any fears cause you constant anxiety?	____
Do your fears interfere with your sleep?	____

accomplish far more in a given time than you thought possible; fear can help you focus on what's important in life. Fear is capable of all this because it sharpens your senses and makes you acutely aware of what's going on around you and within your body as well. Fear is an emotion, but unlike all other emotions— like sadness, happiness, worry, and anger—it's neither intrinsically negative nor positive. Rather, fear puts the onus on you to make a decision about how to process it and what to do with it.

In the past, whenever the feeling of fear overcame me, I would withdraw, often not following through with my intended action. My fear of failure and disappointing others kept me docile—and out of contention. I continually played the "What if . . .?" game in my mind, and I always lost. "What if I cannot afford my monthly mortgage payments?" "What if I never end up with a job I enjoy?" For many people, the fear of losing their job, their house, or their dignity keeps them, paradoxically, teetering on the edge of those fears being realized, while preventing them from imagining, let alone achieving, their true goals.

But what are you going to do with that fear? Let it paralyze you, so you fold your tent and wait for the end? No way! Again, reverse the trend and let it energize you to fight these problems.

If we dwelled on our fears, on the possibilities that something bad could/will happen, we'd never leave the house. Instead, we know that's not really an option, so we find a way to get over such minor hurdles as bad traffic and unpleasant employment situations. We can and should treat bigger fears the same way—as if they're impeding us from getting what we truly need in our life; fears that, if not diminished, always prevent us from ever reaching our goals. So let these fears put some energy, rather than dread, into your soul. Realize that they can often signal real dangers or disturbances in and around your life, but rather than becoming immobilized and uncertain by them, turn active and resolute to dampen and expunge them.

Most of all, rather than try to ignore your fears, learn from them. They teach you about yourself, pointing to your weak points and biggest obstacles, and help you map out the most direct route to achieving great levels of happiness and success.

The next step is to **challenge your fears, one by one.** Review the personal fears you wrote down in the self-evaluation, and resolve now to try to prevent them from overwhelming you at any point in your life. Because they're so natural and, unfortunately, taught to us, they will always be knocking on your door. But it's up to you whether or not to let them in, and what to do with them once they're inside.

When faced with a fear I always ask myself, "Why am I afraid? What really is keeping me from reaching my goal?" Instead of examining fears as a group, looking at them one by one makes them more manageable to work through. Usually the fears I have had aren't nearly as bad as I had originally thought. Then direct your energy at each individual fear and, once you have succeeded in defacing its value, move on to the next one. If you fail to conquer a fear, do not get discouraged. Believe that with time and effort you will overcome it—and, know that one stumble does not mean you will stumble dealing with other fears in the future.

Some of your fears will reappear until you've mastered how to handle them. Others will come back no matter what you do, so it may take continual effort throughout your life to keep them in check. Achieving success in the first twelve weeks of this program will help you conquer whatever fears you have by showing you what you're capable of—making you more aware of yourself, mentally and physically, and improving your instincts every step of the way.

Plenty of my clients who I also work with in life coaching had previously failed at one small piece of their goal and would give up without trying another path or redirecting their energy. Why? They feared more failure if they moved forward, so a minor failure kept the larger, more rewarding goals from occurring. For instance, a client of mine did not apply to a graduate program, even after spending months getting all the necessary information and applications; though she was more than qualified, she was afraid they would not accept her. After working with me and dealing with her fear of rejection, she managed to summon up the courage to apply the next semester and was accepted without a problem.

Never give up, no matter what fears and letdowns transpire. Prepare yourself, emotionally and intuitively, so that previous goal killers—negative thoughts, negative people, and negative situations—can no longer determine what you can or cannot achieve. Trust your gut, and the end result will be in your favor.

Last, you must **face your fears with courage.** Have you ever wanted something so badly that, even though you were afraid, you went ahead and tried for it anyway? Like skydiving out of an airplane, or asking someone out on a date when you weren't sure what the answer would be? For instance, I am terrified of heights, especially when I had to cross the aluminum ladders that were tied together across the enormous crevasses of Everest's Khumbu icefall. But that was the only route to the summit, so I could either confront my acrophobia or see my goal of reaching the summit vanish in the Himalayan wind. What I did was use the fear coursing through my body to focus intensely on each ladder rung. If you haven't dealt with your fears directly, now is the time. Tell yourself, "I am going to do it!"

From now on, whenever you're presented with fear, immediately think of it as a challenge to work through (positive); next, proceed without hesitation (face fear), without looking back or too far forward, and stay in the moment (instinct), which is when you can defeat fear. There is no goal that you cannot accomplish once you have learned how to overcome fear.

For every one reason not to follow your dreams, there are at least two other reasons to do so—so don't erase the dreams from your mind before they are given a chance to be realized. As you go through the following months of Hyperfitness, watch each day for signs of fears that are holding you back. Write down any fears you may have had that day before turning in for the night. Then the next morning, read over what you wrote, and try not to let those fears keep you from achieving your tasks for the day. Face at least one of those fears within the coming week and conquer it with the lessons applied in this program.

Because the variety of drills and exercises—along with variations in repetitions, rep tempo, weight amounts, and heart rate training sectors—keep your body guessing, your muscles and joints probably become sore after workouts. This is a good thing, because your body isn't settling into a plateau, unlike what happens in many other programs at this point. Meanwhile, no matter how demanding the workout feels, you should also notice that your overall recovery

BODY CHECK

Taking Stock (Weeks 5 and 6)

If you've consistently followed this program for a month, you will have noticed some significant developments in your body: namely, less fat and more lean muscle, along with greater athleticism that extends to any activity you do, from picking up a child to swinging a golf club. Your hard work is creating encouraging results, so I hope your motivation level remains high.

time is improving. Applying the Hyperfare guidelines will boost your recovery levels and subsequent energy.

Hyperfare Carbohydrates

"Ah, here we go. Now I get to find out what I can't eat." Did I catch you thinking that? If so, I don't blame you, as most fitness and diet books love to go off on carbohydrates, essentially blaming them for the obesity epidemic.

Well, that's bollocks. In Hyperfitness, you may end up consuming more carbohydrates than ever before if you're putting the calorie-crushing Hyperstrength workouts into practice. You're now training like an athlete, and an athlete requires fuel for his or her muscles; so while protein helps repair the muscles and fat can lend satiety to the meals, carbohydrates provide the main source of energy. Sit down at any training table with a bunch of rowers, rock climbers, or soccer players—who all possess prized athletic physiques—and you'll see them plow through the carbohydrates. They're not eating massive amounts of protein and holding off on the bread; if they did, they'd see their performance drop significantly. In fact, they'd probably bonk well before reaching the finish line or the end of the match!

I'm not telling you to go out and start devouring huge plates of pasta after your training session. Because you're probably not working out for the two-plus hours that most highly trained athletes are, you also don't need the second plate of spaghetti. But the first plate? Go for it!

The problem isn't carbohydrates in general, but the *kind* of carbohydrates that are consumed. I want you to essentially abandon high-glycemic, refined carbohydrates and eat unrefined, **low-glycemic carbohydrates**. The glycemic index (GI) ranks foods by how they affect our blood sugar levels in the two to three hour period after eating. High-GI foods are rapidly digested and absorbed, causing blood sugar spikes as well as increased appetite; low-GI foods take longer to digest and produce slow rises in blood sugar and insulin levels, which provides an even flow of energy, makes you less likely to store food as fat, and lowers your overall hunger levels.

If you pay attention to how food affects your hunger level, the GI may start to click. Most fruit, for example, is very low on the scale, so that's why a single apple can be a fulfilling snack. Conversely, a sandwich on white bread (high-GI) is far less satisfying for your appetite than one on whole-grain bread; similarly, juices (very high-GI) barely register in your stomach, while a piece of fruit does.

The GI, however, is not the only barometer to follow when choosing your carbohydrates. You also should eat **"clean" carbohydrates**, which aren't chock-full of saturated fats, oils, and calories. That means eating foods such as french fries, chips, onion rings, doughnuts, bagels, cookies, and cakes on an extremely limited basis.

You also want to go with carbohydrates that simply have more nutrition per calorie than other forms, so choose **complex carbohydrates.** They are full of fiber, vitamins, and minerals that take longer to digest in the body than other carbohydrates—and they're good for keeping your metabolism burning efficiently. In fact, the fiber in vegetables, fruits, and whole grains has been proven to lower the risk of heart disease, according to a recent study in the *American Journal of Clinical Nutrition.* Whole-grain bread, steel-cut oats, whole-wheat pasta, brown rice, vegetables, beans, and nuts are all complex carbohydrates. Ideally you should try to eat **organic** (so you're not ingesting any pesticide residue or genetically engineered foods) and produce **grown locally** (which ensures a higher nutrition content because the food is considerably fresher), meaning within 150 miles.

Carbohydrates should play a significant role in your eating habits as you transform your life to Hyperfitness. Carbohydrates are the finest resource of quick energy, and clean carbohydrates are some of the healthiest foods you can consume. Without them, your exercise and energy levels will dwindle, and your ability to stay with the program will be seriously compromised.

What do I suggest for carbohydrate consumption levels? Since Trekkers are exercising for at least a half hour a day, five days a week, at moderate to intense levels, they should strive for an intake of 3 to 4 grams of carbohydrates per pound of body weight. Climbers and Sherpas will require slightly more because of the increased exercise time and a higher metabolism.

Hyperstrength, Phase Three:
Weeks 5 and 6

You've arrived at Week 5, so congratulations. Many others never reach this week. You are different, and you are succeeding. You've overcome huge obstacles to get his far and have learned many valuable things about yourself along the way.

At this stage of the Hyperstrength program, all levels will focus on power development: building explosiveness, force, and cardiovascular and muscular strength. While the cardiovascular training for Trekkers will develop more stamina, remaining near their aerobic threshold for longer durations, their continued circuit training will produce more overall strength. Trekkers will decrease their total exercise time slightly as they increase the weight they push or pull.

Meanwhile, the cardiovascular regimen for Climbers and Sherpas will emphasize speed, while increasing their weight by at least 15 percent. While Climbers and Trekkers will take the weekend off to promote active recovery,

Stay Away from Low-Carb Trends

The fact that you hear about low-carb dieting less and less tells you it not only doesn't work in the long term, but also is not beneficial to your health. In the short term, it can result in weight loss because these low-carb plans cut hundreds of calories from your daily allotment. Of course, the weight that comes off is mostly muscle, and any fat lost comes right back as soon as you introduce carbohydrates back into the system (low-carbing creates a condition called ketogenesis, when the body literally thinks it's starving—nice, huh?). And your ability to exercise is significantly decreased, simply because the stored energy in your muscles comes from carbohydrates, not bacon and steaks.

Another ridiculous trend is tracking "net carbs," which are supposedly found by subtracting the carbohydrates that do not affect blood sugar levels—such as fiber, natural sugar, and alcohols—from the total carbohydrates of a particular food. Not only has/did (it's a fast-dying trend, thank God) this produce some awful food, it didn't work. The bottom line is that net carbohydrates do not take away calories or hide carbohydrates from your diet.

Hyperfitness nutrition is not about starving yourself, pushing the carbohydrates off your plate, or going to bed hungry. It's about healthy, all-natural, organic, life-sustaining, quality eating for a lifetime. The Hyperfare suggestions enable you to eat more, have more energy, and feel alive!

Sherpas will be asked to exercise on at least one of the weekend days in conjunction with their active recovery day.

You should now be thinking about your short-term goals daily to enforce the idea that your Inner Everest and short-term goals are plausible. You've come this far, so do not let the mental preparation and weeks of hard work go to waste. Stay on your toes!

Breathing, the Right Way

SECRET SUMMIT TIP

To get the maximum from your workout and to help make your day less stressful, you must breathe properly: from the belly! In other words, see your abdomen rise before your chest does. Place your hand on your belly, right below the navel, and pay close attention to the rise and fall of your abdominal cavity. When you take shallow breaths during exercise, carbon dioxide gathers in your bloodstream, which can affect your performance level, hence your strength and focus levels.

When I run, one of the several methods I use to maintain a nice tempo is to breathe at my pace and in rhythm with my running. It usually consists of one breath (within two strides) and three continuous exhales with my running stride. This assures me that I am exhaling and inhaling at a constant rate. Even on hill runs and anaerobic sessions, I breathe the same way to fool my body into thinking it's still the same pace, thus expanding my muscle endurance. Breathing this way helps preserve the energy storage within, and I am able to go longer while building oxygen and lung

capacity strength. The rhythm pattern can be whatever works for you. The important thing is to find it, and then see how it works for you. Try a two/two, two/one, and so on.

I also find that a few deep breaths from the diaphragm during my runs also proves useful. Most people use a shallow breath from their chest, which leaves a lot of unused breathing space in your body. With that in mind, for one training session I will breathe deeply—with long inhales and long exhales—while running at a moderately challenging pace. Try to maintain these long breaths until you can't do it anymore, then slow your pace and breathe normally again before resuming the exercise.

Complete exhalation exercises also work well. Do an Inner Everest drill until you are out of breath, then stop and take deep breaths with full exhalations, making sure there is not one ounce of O_2 left in your lungs. Repeat three times. Start back with a light jog and then resume the drill soon after.

Maria T., Thirty-four, Elementary School Teacher

"I've never felt that I've been athletic. In fact, growing up I was always chosen last for team sports. Sean's programs have challenged me to do my best, become physically fit, and they have instilled confidence in my own abilities. Through Sean, I have learned that determination and hard work will drive you to do your best in all areas of your life."

Charles P., Jr., Twenty-six, Chief Operating Officer

"Before I began Sean's Hyperfitness program, I weighed 230 pounds. I could barely run three miles without getting extremely winded and fatigued. I had no real physical or personal goals. I was lazy and could care less about my diet. As time went by, the pounds kept adding up and my clothes got tighter and tighter. I knew that I had to make a change.

"I joined Sean's Hyperfitness program in December 2005. I was out of shape and had a hard time keeping up with the rest of his students. I could have easily dropped out, but Sean was extremely motivating and encouraged me to stick to his program and promised that results would come.

"A crucial component of Sean's program is setting personal fitness goals that at the time seem unattainable. Meanwhile, Sean was leading an expedition to Mount Kilimanjaro in May 2006. I've always enjoyed hiking, and climbing a mountain in my physical condition seemed impossible at the time. I decided to make the Kilimanjaro climb my first Inner Everest goal! Setting such a lofty goal gave meaning and purpose to my workouts. I found that I was getting stronger faster and pushing myself harder and harder in class. All the while I was following Sean's recommendations on healthy eating habits. Pretty soon my pants started getting looser, my energy levels increased, and I had a renewed outlook on life and especially fitness. I actually enjoyed exercising! In May 2006 I reached my goal, and climbed Mount Kilimanjaro with Sean.

"Today, at 195 pounds, I continue to set new and exciting fitness and personal goals for myself. I recently competed in my first 20K and completed the run in less than one hour and thirty minutes. As further testament to the Hyperfitness program, I competed in my first 50K within my first year of the Hyperfitness experience. Most important, I enjoy sharing my newfound love of fitness with my children, and my wife and I now enjoy our weekend trail runs together. My outlook on life, and on setting and attaining goals, has completely changed in less than a year."

TREKKER ▲ Weeks 5 and 6 • Monday/Wednesday/Friday

Go straight through the 6 drills below, 3 times, with 1½ to 2 minutes rest between each complete round of exercises. Increase the weight 10 percent after the first Monday and Wednesday sessions for a power push, and decrease the drill time from 1 minute to 45 seconds. If you exhaust your muscles before the time is up, then take a brief rest before finishing the set.

1. **Push-up with Resistance Band,** 10 reps (do the push-up on your knees if needed), **to Quick Jumps with Medicine Ball over Band,** 20 reps; repeat the series until 1½ minutes are up
2. **Squat Medicine Ball Underhand Throw Jump to Self-Catch**
3. **Medicine Ball Squat Jump Throw, to Catch, to Medicine Ball Straight-Arm Twist**
4. **Medicine Ball Jumping Jack,** 10 reps, **to 1–4 Box Drill with Medicine Ball,** 10 reps; repeat the series until 1½ minutes are up
5. **Inverted V**
6. **Squat Jump to Reverse Grip Pull-up**

IE Drill: Go straight through the 3 drills with little to no rest between them; for each drill, go 25 yards down and back; repeat the round 4 more times, again with as little rest as possible (H.E.S. 2–4).

1. **Knee Highs**
2. **Upright Crab Walk**
3. **2 Lunges to 1 Frog Jump**

Stretch (see pages 58–59)

Push-up with Resistance Band to Quick Jumps with Medicine Ball over Band: Get into push-up position, holding a resistance band around your shoulder blades over your back and held taut under each hand on the ground. After 10 push-ups, jump your feet under your chest and grab the medicine ball and put the band on the floor. Bring the medicine ball to your chest and jump side-to-side over the band.

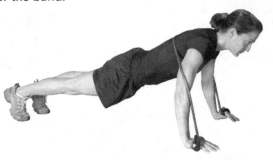

Squat Medicine Ball Underhand Throw Jump to Self-Catch: Take a wide stance with your feet pointed out slightly and hold the medicine ball between your legs. Squat down, and then on the way up throw the medicine ball vertically up while jumping off the ground. Catch underhanded and repeat.

Medicine Ball Squat Jump Throw, to Catch, to Medicine Ball Straight-Arm Twist: Squat down with the medicine ball at chest height, palms facing up holding the medicine ball, then jump up while throwing the ball upward. Catch the ball and hold it straight out in front of you for left and right twists.

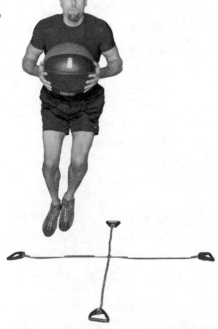

Medicine Ball Jumping Jack to 1–4 Box Drill with Medicine Ball: Begin jumping jacks with medicine ball at chest level. When your legs go out, bring the medicine ball above your head. For the box drill, use rope or tape to cross 2 lines on the floor. Hop clockwise around the box, and then counterclockwise while holding the medicine ball at chest level.

Inverted V: Start in modified push-up position with your glutes in the air so your body forms an inverted V. Keep your legs straight and stand on your toes, then bend your elbows while lowering your head and shoulders toward the floor. Go down until your forehead lightly touches floor, and then push back up.

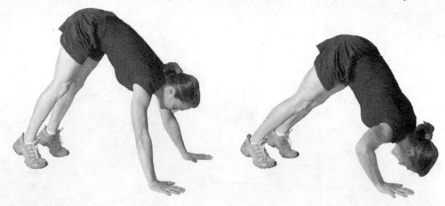

Squat Jump to Reverse Grip Pull-up: Squat down under a pull-up bar and explode up to grab the bar with an underhand or reverse grip. Do a complete pull-up, then come down for another squat.

Knee Highs: Run while bringing knee to chest with each stride.

Upright Crab Walk: Walk forward in a squat position, with your hands on top of your head.

Lunge: Stand with your hands on your hips, then take 2 large steps forward by having the lead leg descend until the thigh is almost parallel to the ground, while the back knee almost touches the ground. Make sure the lead knee never goes beyond the perpendicular line formed by the lead toes.

Frog Jump: With your hands on top of your head, squat down to 90 degrees with your legs and rise, hopping forward, two feet at a time.

TREKKER ▲ Weeks 5 and 6 • Tuesday/Thursday

This workout requires access to a stationary bike or elliptical machine. If you are outside, select a trail or grass to run on that ideally has some hilly qualities. At any time during the session, sing one song as loud as you can while keeping an aerobic cadence.

1. Warm up 5 minutes starting slow and building to a moderate pace (H.E.S. 1–2)
2. 1 minute sustained effort at as close to AT (anaerobic threshold) as possible with medium resistance on your equipment of choice, 45 seconds easy; 4 reps total (H.E.S. 2 on recovery)
3. **Diagonal Jumps** in 1–4 Box; 5 reps (H.E.S. 3)
4. 1 minute sustained push near AT with medium resistance, then 45 seconds easy; repeat the series 4 times (H.E.S. 2 on recovery)
5. **Hands-Down to Up Squat Jump,** 5 reps, **to Full Jumping Jacks,** 5 reps, **to Cross-Country,** 6 reps; do the series 8 times total (H.E.S. 3–4)
6. Jump Rope, 1 minute and 15 seconds skipping rope fast, then 15 second rest; repeat 8 minutes; put a picture of a goal on the wall in front of you (H.E.S. 3–4)

Core: Bicycles, 3 sets, 20 times; Downward-Facing Dog Pose after each set of bicycles, hold for 20 seconds

Stretch (see pages 58–59)

Diagonal Jumps in 1–4 Box: Make 4 boxes with 2 crossed bands or jump ropes. Jump so you land in each of the 4 boxes once each rep, such as 1 to 3 to 2 to 4, for 12 reps (jumps); complete 5 various combinations.

Hands-Down to Up Squat Jump, to Full Jumping Jacks, to Cross-Country: Reach down in a squat position touching the floor with the palms of your hands up, then jump straight up as high as you can and, reaching up as high as you can, immediately perform a Full Jumping Jack, page 97; Cross-Country, page 98

Bicycles: Lie on your back on the ground. While using a slow bicycling motion with your legs (making sure to extend each leg fully and bring opposite knee to mid-body), do a crossover crunch and bring one elbow to the opposite knee.

Downward-Facing Dog Pose: Start on your hands and knees with your back flat and head in line with your back. Curl your toes under and straighten your legs, and then push upward with your arms. Lengthen your spine while trying to keep your legs straight and feet flat on the ground. Your weight should be evenly distributed between your hands and feet.

CLIMBER ▲▲ Weeks 5 and 6 • Monday/Wednesday/Friday

In the following 4 drills, you will perform a set of the first exercise (which is sometimes two moves combined) and immediately follow with a set of the second exercise. Take a few breaths, then repeat each drill twice more. After the 3 sets of each drill, rest for at least 2 minutes before moving to the next one. (Note: Increase the time duration to complete most exercises due to increase in chosen weight, by *15 percent*, established in first Monday and Wednesday sessions.)

1A. Incline Clap Push-up, 3 reps, to **Jump over Step,** 10 reps
1B. Spider Tip to Rings/Bar/Straps Pull-up, 15 reps

2A. Dumbbell Push-up to Straight-up Dumbbell Jump, 15 reps
2B. Cable Squat Jump, 20 reps

3A. Staggered Push-up, 14 reps (7 reps each side), **to Triceps Forearm Push-up,** 5 reps; repeat the series twice (to exhaustion if reps cannot be met)
3B. Cable Squat, to Cable Row Hold, to Low Squat Row Hold, 12 reps

4A. Straddle Step Dumbbell Squat, to Jump on Step, to Press Overhead, 10 reps
4B. Heavy Medieval Bastard Full Crunch to Touch Toes, 25 reps

IE Drill 1: 30 yards up, 30 yards back, 2 times each stage (H.E.S. 3–4). Rest 1 minute before continuing to IE Drill 2.

  1. Evolution of Frog Jump; 4 stages, up and back

IE Drill 2: 30 yards up, 30 yards back, 4 times (H.E.S. 3–4).

1. **Split Squats with Medicine Ball Between Legs**
2. **Medicine Ball Monkey Arms Run**
3. **Squat Jump Forward with Medicine Ball Toss Front and Back**

Repeat the entire series again if time and schedule allow.

Downward-Facing Dog Pose: Hold for 20 seconds

Stretch (see pages 58–59)

Incline Clap Push-up to Jump over Step: Using a step with at least 5 risers, get into push-up position, with your hands on the step and feet on the floor. Explode out of third clap push-up, then pop your feet up to just in front of the step, and then jump forward over step. Turn around and repeat.

Spider Tip to Rings/Bar/Straps Pull-up: Start with your feet together and your body in crouch position with your fingertips touching the floor on the outside of your feet. Shoot your feet out behind you, then pop your feet back to start position. Jump to execute a pull-up with your palms facing in, slow on the lowering phase of pull-up.

Dumbbell Push-up to Straight-up Dumbbell Jump: Do a dumbbell push-up (do a full push-up with each hand wrapped around a dumbbell handle), then pop your feet under your chest and jump up while holding your dumbbells by your sides.

Cable Squat Jump: Hold the cable handle from a cable machine at mid-height behind your back with both hands, then squat jump forward. Step back, and repeat as fast as possible.

Staggered Push-up to Triceps Forearm Push-up: Do staggered push-ups (placing one hand near rib cage and the other closer to shoulder), then place your hands in front of your head and bring your forearms to touch the floor, performing a triceps push-up.

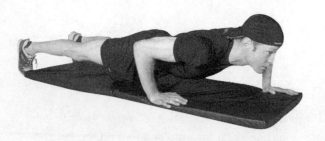

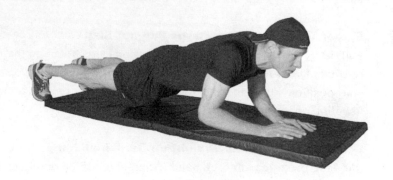

Cable Squat, to Cable Row Hold, to Low Squat Row Hold: Hold the cables
at high level, then squat down while pulling the cables toward you. Hold squat
and cable row position with your elbows as far back as possible, and flex your
biceps for 1 second. Then bring your glutes to your ankles (keeping your heels
on ground), while still keeping an isometric hold with the cable row. (In an
isometric hold, there is no movement; muscles contract but do not shorten.)
Next, squat back up and extend your arms at the top.

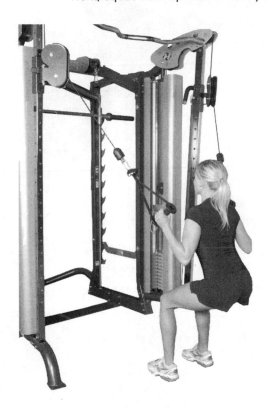

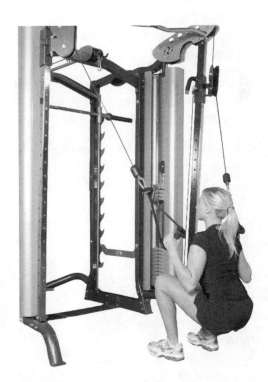

Straddle Step Dumbbell Squat, to Jump on Step, to Press Overhead: Stand straddling an elevated step, with at least 5 risers, with a dumbbell in each hand at shoulder level (with palms facing in), and squat down until your glutes touch the step. Then jump onto the step and press the dumbbells overhead.

Heavy Medieval Bastard Full Crunch to Touch Toes: Lie on your back on the floor with your hands holding an extra-heavy medicine ball behind your head and your legs extended straight in front of you 2 feet off the floor. Do a full crunch, bending your legs, having the medicine ball touch your toes.

Evolution of Frog Jump: 1) Maintaining a squat position, walk forward 2) frog jump (with hands placed on top of your head and your feet slightly angled out, squat down until your glutes are almost near your ankles and your knees go out in the same angle as your toes; then explode forward, jumping like a frog), 3) feet-together frog jump hop, 4) feet-wide-to-feet-closed frog jump hop.

Split Squats with Medicine Ball Between Legs: Do split squats forward while bringing the medicine ball underneath your lead leg during each split squat forward, as fast as possible.

Medicine Ball Monkey Arms Run: Move forward keeping the medicine ball between your legs, switching arms from one side to the other with each forward step, making sure the medicine ball does not touch the floor.

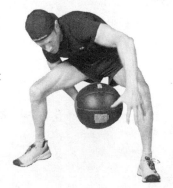

Squat Jump Forward with Medicine Ball Toss Front and Back: Hold the medicine ball between your legs with both hands reaching out behind you. As you squat jump forward switch your hands around to the front and catch the medicine ball between your legs before it touches the ground. Squat jump forward again and switch your hands to behind you and catch the medicine ball between your legs before it touches the ground.

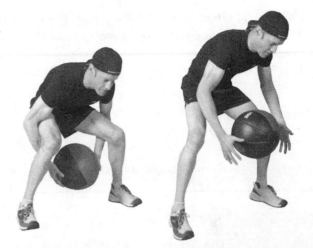

CLIMBER ▲▲ Weeks 5 and 6 • Tuesday/Thursday

This workout requires access to a trail or grass (preferably with some hilly areas) outside or a treadmill. Time yourself and work through the workout as quickly and safely as possible; track your length of time for the complete routine each workout session, as building speed and progression is the goal. If you must stop early because of time and schedule restraints, do so.

1. 1 mile outside or on treadmill at 2% incline, holding medicine ball (at chest height)
2. **Medicine Ball Jumping Jack,** 20 reps (big breath)
3. Repeat **Medicine Ball Jumping Jacks**
4. Treadmill: 2 minute run at 15% incline
5. 1 minute walk at 15% incline
6. 2 minute run at 12% incline
7. 1 minute walk at 12% incline
8. 4 minute run at 3% incline
9. **Medicine Ball Jump on Bosu to Medicine Ball Slam,** 20 reps
10. **Spread-Eagle Jump with Medicine Ball,** 10 reps
11. Repeat 1–10 one more time (H.E.S. 2–4).
12. **The Straw,** 2 minute walk at 3% incline

Core: Rock the Cradle, 3 sets, 20 times, to 1 Full Standing Extension; hold for 10 seconds between each set

Stretch (see pages 58–59)

Medicine Ball Jumping Jack: Do a regular jumping motion with your feet, while bringing the medicine ball from chest to overhead with every jump.

Medicine Ball Jump on Bosu to Medicine Ball Slam: Hold the medicine ball at your chest and jump onto the Bosu and off to the other side. Then slam the medicine ball on the floor. Repeat back and forth from side to side with a medicine ball slam on each side.

Spread-Eagle Jump with Medicine Ball: With the medicine ball at your chest, squat and jump, spreading your legs out while bringing the medicine ball overhead and then back to your chest upon landing on your feet.

The Straw: Plug your nose and breathe only through a straw. If you become dizzy, immediately remove straw and breathe normally.

Rock the Cradle to 1 Full Standing Extension: Lie on your back on a mat with your legs extended straight and your feet off the floor with your arms extended behind your head and off the floor. Rock forward and back without your hands or feet touching the mat. Then interlace your fingers and stretch your body completely overhead.

SHERPA ▲▲▲ **Weeks 5 and 6** · **Monday/Wednesday/Friday**

In the 3 intense drills that follow, you will perform a set of the first exercise (which is sometimes two moves combined), then immediately follow with a set of the second exercise and then a third exercise. Take a few deep breaths, then repeat each drill twice more. After the 3 sets of each drill, rest for at least 2 minutes (or the time it takes to organize equipment for the next drill) before moving to the next one. (Note: Increased time duration is to be expected to complete most exercises because of the increase in chosen weight [*15 percent*] established in the first Monday and Wednesday sessions.)

1A **Upside-Down Bosu Show-Hand Push-ups with 3-Point Position,** 16 reps or at least 1 minute

1B. **Heavy Medieval Bastard Squat Jump Throw and Catch to Jump Slams,** 15 reps

1C. **Barbell Squat Row, to Throw Release and Catch, to Press Overhead in Front,** 15 reps

2A. **Underhand Grip Pull-ups with Rings/Straps/Bar to Each Above Hand,** 12 reps

2B. **Triceps Push-up on Medicine Ball,** 3 reps, **to Jump Medicine Ball Daffies,** 2 reps, **to Jump with Medicine Ball Overhead,** 1 rep; perform series 10 times

2C. **Lying Dumbbell Twist** (each side = 1 rep), 30 reps

3A. **Feet Together Back to Front,** 5 reps, **to Full Bar Spin, to Pull-up** with 2-second isometric hold at top; perform series 10 times

3B. **180-Degree Jumps on Step with Dumbbells,** 20 reps

3C. **Dumbbell Squat Row Switch Catches,** 50 reps

IE Drill 1: Repeat the series 4 times. Rest is limited to no more than 30 seconds at any one time (H.E.S. 3–4).

1. **Single Leg Broad Jump to Single Leg Zigzag Jump,** 40 yards (20 yards each leg), 2 reps
2. **Crocodile Walk, to Stiff-Arm Crawl, to Full Jumping Jack,** 20 yards, 2 reps
3. **One-Arm Scale the Whale,** up and back, 20 yards, 2 reps

IE Drill 2: Have 2 steps or obstacles lined up one in front of the other; use 1–5 risers for height. Repeat the series 4 times. Rest is limited to no more than 30 seconds at any one time.

1. **Knee Highs over Steps,** 10 reps (up and back = 1 rep)
2. **Feet Together Jump over Steps,** first side-to-side, then up and back while still facing front, 10 reps (up and back = 1 rep)

Downward-Facing Dog Pose: Hold for 20 seconds

Stretch (see pages 58–59)

Upside-Down Bosu Show-Hand Push-ups with 3-Point Position: Turn Bosu upside-down and get into push-up position with one hand placed in middle of the Bosu and the other hand on the floor, while placing the foot on the same side as the Bosu off the floor. As you rise from each push-up, lift up the hand that is on the floor and show your palm out. Switch feet after 8 reps.

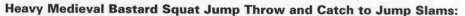

Heavy Medieval Bastard Squat Jump Throw and Catch to Jump Slams: With an extra-heavy medicine ball at chest level, squat down and throw it upward on way up. Jump up and catch the ball while it's overhead and then slam it to the ground.

Barbell Squat Row, to Throw Release and Catch, to Press Overhead in Front: Place one end of a barbell against the wall and put both hands on the other, weighted end. Squat and row, bringing barbell toward your chest, at same

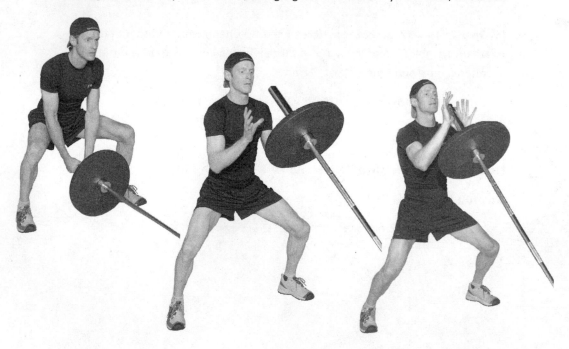

time, then throw the bar upward and catch it, palms up and near shoulder level. Press overhead in front of your head.

Underhand Grip Pull-ups with Rings/Straps/Bar to Each Above Hand:
Take an underhand (palms facing you) grip with rings/straps/bar and execute a pull-up with your chin rising above and over each hand.

Triceps Push-up on Medicine Ball, to Jump Medicine Ball Daffies, to Jump with Medicine Ball Overhead: Put both hands on the medicine ball and do a triceps push-up, bringing your solar plexus to your hands. Pop your feet to under your chest and grab the medicine ball with your hands, then jump upward daffy-style (scissorslike position) holding the medicine ball, and then squat jump holding the medicine ball above your head.

Lying Dumbbell Twist: Lie on your back with your legs bent and feet off the floor, and both hands around the dumbbell with your arms bent. Twist the dumbbell from one side to the other, touching the floor.

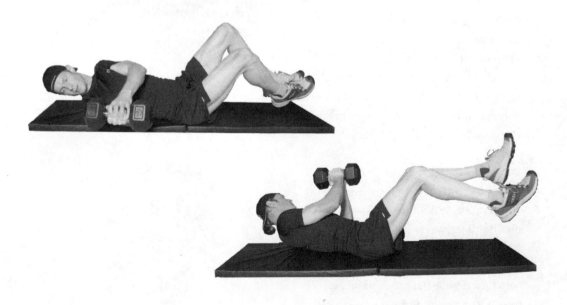

Feet Together Back to Front, to Full Bar Spin, to Pull-up: With your hands in push-up position and your legs straight and feet together, jump your feet to under your chest and back out 5 times. Then squat jump to an overhand grab of a pull-up bar/strap/ rings and do a full body spin, bringing your legs between your arms and then turning your body over. Follow with a pull-up with 2-second isometric hold at top.

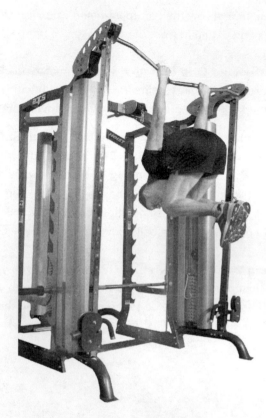

180-Degree Jumps on Step with Dumbbells: With dumbbells at shoulder height, stand next to a step with at least 5 risers. Step on the step with the foot nearest and your body facing sideways. Do a 180-degree jump spin and land with the other foot now on the step, and repeat.

Dumbbell Squat Row Switch Catches: Stand with legs shoulder-width apart, holding a dumbbell with one hand between your legs. Perform squat. As you rise from the squat, pull the dumbbell straight up and release, catching it with the other hand, and return to a squat. Repeat on opposite side after each rep.

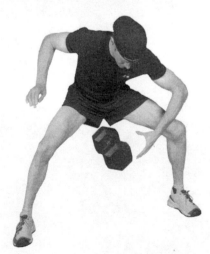

Single Leg Broad Jump to Single Leg Zigzag Jump: Jump off and land on one leg only, then do single leg diagonal jumps back.

Crocodile Walk, to Stiff-Arm Crawl, to Full Jumping Jack: With your arms bent and your body in push-up position, "walk" forward without bending your legs and staying on your toes for 10 yards. Next, straighten your arms and go forward dragging your legs for 10 yards. Last, do full jumping jacks while moving forward 20 yards.

One-Arm Scale the Whale: With 1 hand on a towel placed on a hard court or smooth surface, get into a running back set position, and run forward.

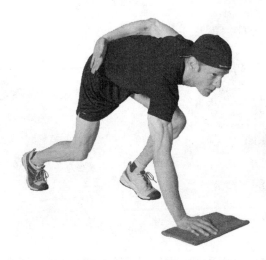

Knee Highs over Steps: Jog, bringing knees as high as possible, up and back.

Feet Together Jump over Steps: With your feet together, jump diagonally over steps with at least 3 risers. Then with your body still facing forward, jump diagonally back.

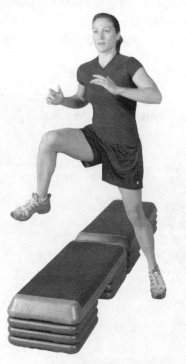 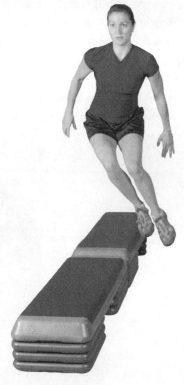

SHERPA ▲▲▲ Weeks 5 and 6 • Tuesday/Thursday

Time yourself and work through the workout as quickly and safely as possible, tracking the length of time for rounds each workout session—building speed and progression is the goal. H.E.S. 2–4.

1. Squat and jump while throwing the medicine ball up the wall, 10 reps, then hold your breath and run with the medicine ball across a basketball court or 25 yards (don't blow out air until you've reached the end line), then on your back to roll up, pick up the medicine ball, and jump straight up with the medicine ball overhead, 10 reps. Then hold your breath and run back with the medicine ball (up and back = 1 round); perform 7 rounds

2. Treadmill: 3% incline for 5 minutes at hard pace (just below AT)

3. **Rock Climber,** 4 reps, to Knuckle to Hand Push-up, 4 reps; perform 4 times

4. 15% incline speed walk for 5 minutes

5. **Rock Climber,** 4 reps, to Knuckle to Hand Push-up, 4 reps; perform 4 times

6. 3% for 5 minutes at hard pace (just below AT)

7. **Rock Climber,** 4 reps, to Knuckle to Hand Push-up, 4 reps; perform 4 times

8. 15% incline speed walk for 5 minutes

9. **Rock Climber,** 4 reps, to Knuckle to Hand Push-up, 4 reps; perform 4 times

10. Repeat 1–9 one more round (H.E.S. 3–4)

IE Drill: Jump rope, 3-pound rope, one song, resting only when very necessary (H.E.S. 3–4) **The Straw:** With treadmill, walk at 6% incline or cycle on bike at low resistance with consistent cadence for 3–5 minutes, plugging the nose and breathing only through a straw. If you become dizzy, immediately remove straw and breathe normally.

Core: Crunch Throw Heavy Medieval Bastard: Lie on your back holding heavy medicine ball, and crunch upward, releasing ball above chest. Clap 2 times and catch ball on its desent. 30 reps, 2 deep breaths; repeat

Stretch (see pages 58–59)

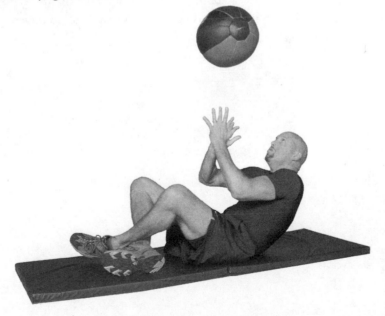

Rock Climber: Get into push-up position. Keeping your upper body fixed, bring your right knee to your chest, then straight again; left knee to chest and straight again; right foot straight out to 3 o'clock and back again; left foot straight out to 9 o'clock and back again. Do this in a staccato, bouncy rhythm.

Knuckle to Hand Push-up: In push-up position, do a knuckle push-up (on your knuckles instead of your hands) and then jump your hands to a regular push-up.

SHERPA   ▲▲▲   Weeks 5 and 6 • Weekend

Hike for at least 2 hours on Saturday or Sunday, carrying a load of at least 30 pounds in your rucksack. For weight, buy bags of sand or rice. Place the rice or sand in zip-top bags, and organize appropriately in the rucksack for even weight distribution. During the hike, you should try to maintain a steady pace without stopping to rest. Make sure you have water and a gel/energy bar available to eat and drink on the go. Do not worry about your heart rate, and just try to maintain a steady pace for at least 2 hours. Your other weekend day should be active recovery (see Appendix D).

Chapter 6

LINKING LADDERS

Weeks 7 and 8

WE ARE ALL, AT THE CORE, CLIMBERS. Climbing is the ultimate metaphor in life, just as falling is a metaphor for losing one's way toward a goal. These metaphors aptly describe the inevitable peaks and valleys of existence. We fall off the wagon, fall into debt, try to climb out of it, trip over obstacles, find our footing, land on our feet, and so on. It's remarkable how entrenched these phrases are in our English vocabulary.

Like the mountain climber, we must deal with conditions that shift constantly, like the wind, and conditions that rise and fall, like the sun. These conditions include our relations with family members and work mates, financial concerns, work pressure, health crises, and troubling news—to say nothing about taking care of the kids, getting in the workout, preparing healthy meals, and doing the errands. Of course, *how* we deal with them is what separates the exceptional climber from the stumbling one.

To make your climb a success, you have to find a way to link all of the elements in your life together—including the ones that may seem negative on the surface. To become a complete person who can see the world as a whole, learn to link your love life, your family, your friends, your job, your religion, your workout, your meals, your health, your community, and your world.

I ask you to not only bring all of these elements together, but to inject each with passion. And if you are not able to do so, then you must question whether or not that element—a job, a person, a frequent situation—belongs in your life.

For me, my family, the mountains, Hyperstrength classes and my students, my own Hyperstrength workouts, martial arts, Hyperfare eating, and meditating are the elements that make up my day—they connect me to the world. When they remain linked, I have a beautiful day; when they break apart, I feel incomplete and unsettled.

Linking everything in your life with passion may be the single greatest lesson to learn from this book. It's amazing how much energy and power you can create within yourself by doing such an exercise. If you're able to remain linked, a multitude of wonderful experiences and many great accomplishments await you. Staying on the same page with your every external action and internal thought will start to define you as a person. Others will notice that you speak and move with more purpose, and your destiny for great things will begin to become obvious to others. I call this "linking ladders." Likewise the short-term goals you work toward on your way to reaching your Inner Everest goal should also be linked together to boost your chances of reaching those heights.

Respect your own goals by treating them very seriously and preparing for them thoroughly. Through training your body and your mind with Hyperfitness, you can learn to establish the right links to take you to the desired places in your life and beyond. Integrating all three elements of this program—Hyperstrength, Hypermind, and Hyperfare—into your new lifestyle will create a connection to your goals that is far less likely to be broken.

To assess the strength of your connections, currently, answer these **self-evaluation questions:**

- Do you find it difficult to concentrate or remain energetic if you haven't exercised or eaten a proper meal?
- How do you feel, physically and emotionally, if you haven't exercised?
- How do you feel, physically and emotionally, if you've gone on an eating binge or let a problem get to you?

- Before exercising or facing a dilemma, do you feel happy or sad or nervous? Or do you feel energized?
- How does keeping with daily Hyperstrength training affect the rest of your day, e.g., job, personal life, and so on?
- Have the things you thought were important before beginning the program changed?

See with Your Heart, Not Your Eyes— Your Spiritual Foundation

Having a spiritual foundation can be the key to help you to interrelate everything in your life. If you attach a spiritual foundation to how you think, live, and act, it will help you to see how everything around you is, indeed, connected—as well as how the past can inform your future. Instead of adopting the

Your Touchstone

SECRET SUMMIT TIP

A touchstone is an object that reminds us of a particular moment and keeps us focused on our dreams, and I recommend that you get yourself at least one. Touchstones can help you dispel negative energy, achieve balance, feel love, and find peace of mind. If you do not already have one, select a touchstone during your next self-discovery journey.

I've brought back a touchstone from every major expedition. At home, especially after a particularly stressful day, I like to reach for a rock that I retrieved near the summit of Everest; it reminds me both how far I have come as a person and where I want to be in the future. I picked up the rock near 29,000 feet, on my way down from the summit—and shoved it in my pocket while still trying to maintain a certain mental stability. With its black surface and protruding points smoothed over from time, snow, wind, and other elements, I find

it beautiful. After existing on Everest for thousands, maybe millions, of years, the rock now lives in my home. To me it's a museum artifact that I would not trade for any material possession in the world.

Of course, touchstones do not always have to be rocks! Your touchstone could be a seashell from a magical vacation you took with your spouse or a medal you received for finishing a race. Touchstones will be reference point keepsakes that let you relive your journeys, taking you back to the time when you felt exultant, achieved a goal, or had a memorable experience. So when life throws you a difficult day, pick up your touchstone, close your eyes, take some deep breaths, and let those memories swiftly restore and refresh your strong mind and soul, refocusing you on your future goals.

"woe is me" approach at the first sign of difficulty, believing in a higher power encourages you to delve below the surface of any unfortunate event to learn how it can make you stronger and push you closer to your goals.

I'm not telling you that you must become a follower of an established religion—such as Christianity, Hinduism, Islam, Judaism, Buddhism, or Taoism—in order to fully integrate Hyperfitness into your life. You simply may have a pronounced love for Mother Nature. I encourage you to develop yourself spiritually, because harboring a belief that goes well beyond the self will not only change your approach to life but your outlook as well.

In some ways fitness can be a way to spiritual fulfillment. Instead of an unwanted chore, workouts can become a spiritual route to a calm, centered, and connected self. There is an enormous link between physical output and the mind; both mutually benefit from each other and suffer when one or the other isn't present. My humble hope is that Hyperfitness will make you healthier in body, mind, and spirit—and put you on the path to doing greater things for yourself and many others.

Flowers on the Mountain

TALES FROM THE MOUNTAIN

Each trip to a mountain adds another level to my spiritual foundation. I began climbing mountains because I wanted to stand on the summit and challenge myself, both physically and mentally, but I had no idea of the beauty, nurturing, and life fulfillment that would come from high altitude mountaineering.

In Greenland, I would be on my skis for up to three hours reaching each peak and then heading back to base camp, which left me ample time to experience the majesty of the mountains and such picayune details as the snow bubbles that appeared and popped when my skis cut through them, the white-paste texture of the ice-cap snow, the ever-changing colors of the glacier and sky, and the steady, resonant cadence of my own kick and glide. I was completely connected to nature, and I could see just how essential that connection was to the formation and evolution of the human spirit.

I go on adventures to appreciate the little moments in life that those in high-paced society have a tendency to forget or never experience in the first place: Moments such as the beauty and purity of watching the sun set, holding my wife's hand, hugging my parents, reading a book to my son, seeing a friend smile. Linking all these beautiful moments in life to your dreams will make them more pure and vivid than ever before and, eventually, more fulfilling.

Nature Can Show You What You're Made Of

Through any severe physical test, especially one from Mother Nature, you find out what you're truly made of—which is why I so strongly suggest that you pursue some outdoor short-term goals as a part of this program. Where are you strong, and what part of you is weak? The truth about you is laid bare, and it's a beautiful process. Rather than being a slave to comfort, you will find discomfort both liberating and exhilarating.

These days we spend so much of our time in artificial, climate-controlled environments that it's easy to forget what Mother Nature is really about. For me, being out in the cold, harsh mountain air is exciting because it is so real—and it's especially real when you are moving under your own steam in an environment that you can't reason with. I believe that it connects us with the essential parts of being human. Besides, how can we really understand our role on this earth unless we actually experience it?

Taking a physical and spiritual odyssey will toughen you up. After all, if you had to pick the most consistent trait in those who have accomplished great things, it would probably be being tough. Sticking to the Hyperstrength workouts and Hyperfare nutrition is already toughening you up for the bigger things yet to come.

As long as you stay with it, Hyperfitness can help you achieve great things, in whatever arena you want. Some days you will be sore, so you have to go easier; occasionally you will have to miss a workout, or will consume some food that is definitely not part of Hyperfare—just don't quit. Honestly, if you quit this, then you are quitting life, or at least life at its fullest.

As I tell my clients, if you get through my workouts, the rest of your day will seem like a piece of cake; if you get through each Hyperstrength mini-marathon, you can do anything in life, truly.

Getting Tough on the North Pole

The year after Everest, I decided to compete in the North Pole Marathon—and it was all about toughening up. With mountains, I knew the game, but the Poles were a mystery of nature that I just had to experience. At first, I considered trekking across Antarctica, but then I read about the North Pole Marathon on the Web one day. Never having run a marathon or run in a pair of snowshoes before, I thought it was the perfect challenge for me.

I contacted the organizer, who informed me that several top-level marathoners and arctic explorers were competing. I respected their bios, especially Sir Ranulph Fiennes, called "the greatest living explorer" by Guinness World Record, and who completed seven marathons in seven days all across the globe.

Because of my lack of marathon and arctic experience, I was called the "dark horse" on the marathon's Web site. After injuring my knee two months out from the race, they should have called me the limping pony. Because of the injury, I actually worked out less than usual and did very little specific marathon training. Two weeks before the race, I ran sixteen miles on the treadmill without stopping, and it went better than I expected. When race day arrived, I was excited to go on the strange journey over this frozen land. I didn't have any expectations about winning or losing, but was simply jazzed to be doing a crazy race at the top of the world. If I was going to do well, it'd only be as a result of the Hyperstrength workouts that I'd put myself through for the previous few months—and the fact that my knee felt better. I knew a thing or two about the perilous ice cracks, frostbite, hypothermia, and sub-zero temperatures that I was about to endure, but was admittedly thrown off when the organizer told us about

Hyperfare Fat

The very word *fat* has been demonized across our American food landscape, unlike in many other parts of the world where fat is seen as one of the essential components to the daily diet. Falsely led by so-called experts and diet doctors, we have been told to believe in the literal translation that eating fat makes you fat, and that the only way to lose weight is by eating lean protein and very little fat. (And I forgot to mention: We're also dead wrong, being the fattest nation on earth with the highest rates of heart disease).

In fact, healthy fats do the body tons of good. They give you a concentrated source of energy in the diet and assist in maintaining healthy cell membranes and hormone levels. Healthy fats help with our digestion, expel toxins, and act as lubricants for our joints. These kinds of fats also create satiety by slowing down the threat of polar bear attacks. Russian military men on snowmobiles apparently would protect us from the bears with their guns, but I also noticed that a couple of these "protectors" were consistently drunk.

Because of Everest, I had all the right gear, ankles on up. The snowshoes that a sponsor had given me, however, turned out to be touring snowshoes rather than the running snowshoes that everyone else was wearing. Mine were considerably bigger and more awkward, but I wasn't aware of my equipment deficiency until after the race ended. Later, several of my fellow racers told me they had noticed that I had the wrong snowshoes, but they didn't want to demoralize me just before the starting gun was set to go off.

When it did go off, I hung back to see what kind of pace these guys were going to set. Never having run a marathon before, I really didn't know what I was doing and if anything, felt like I was taking it too easy. Suddenly, after having gone about halfway, I noticed that everybody was starting to fade back. It was at that point that I realized I could actually win this thing. I decided I wasn't about to let anybody pass me. Jumping over ice cracks, keeping my footing through ice floes, and ascending over hills, my only concern was the polar bears, especially during the stretches where nothing or nobody was visible in the white hinterland.

Finally, after three hours and forty-three minutes, I finished and set a new world record. Fiennes was second, thirteen minutes behind me. Victory did taste sweet, but it wasn't the point—I had put my entire Hyperfitness program to the test, and it not only passed but it put me in the winner's circle.

nutrient absorption so you can go longer without feeling hungry, which is critical to the Hyperfare eating style.

The worst fats are hydrogenated fats like margarine and shortening. Just to give you an idea of how unhealthy the process of hydrogenation is, consider that it begins with the cheapest oils—which are usually already rancid, laden with pesticides, or made from genetically engineered crops, or all three!—and then mix them with tiny metal particles. Eventually margarine is produced in form, but not color—its natural color is actually gray, so bleach, dyes, and strong flavors are added to get it to resemble butter.

Partially hydrogenated oils, or trans fats, behave as toxins in our bodies, to the point that our very own cells become partially hydrogenated. This heinous substance has helped contribute to the rise of diseases like cancer, atherosclerosis, diabetes, obesity, and even sterility.

Hyperfare eating includes traditional vegetable oils like extra-virgin olive oil

Sleep

Hyperfitness is intense, but you should never skimp on sleep to fit in your workouts. Lack of sleep is a common problem for the entire developed world, mostly because of technology—cable television, DVD, stereo, and the Internet mean that most people go to bed an hour or more later than they would if they stuck to the traditional book-in-bed routine.

Poor sleep affects nearly everything in your life, including lowering hormone levels (leading to weight gain), high blood pressure, general fatigue, performance decline, brain sluggishness, stress, depression, crankiness, and a compromised immune system.

Many people complain to me that they can put in the seven hours of sleep (I try to aim for between seven and eight hours every night), but it's of the erratic variety. If that describes you, try some of these ways to help create more solid sleep:

- Whatever you do, try not to work out in the late evening. The Hyperstrength workouts should greatly aid your sleep, especially if you do them in the morning.

- Develop a routine in which you eat at the same time each night and go to bed at roughly the same time as well.

- Eat dinner at least two hours before bed in order to prevent acid-reflux from dinner and to simply prevent a digesting stomach from keeping you awake.

- Keep caffeine out of your system from 4 p.m. onward.

- Find out what makes you sleepy (aside from drugs and alcohol), and apply it to your life before bed. For some, reading a book in bed can put them to sleep within minutes; for others, it may backfire and keep them awake for hours. Maybe a warm bath and/or glass of milk (which contains sleep-producing tryptophan) are your sleep tickets. Or, if you're lucky, a love session with your partner can be the trick.

- At least a half hour or more before bed, turn off the brain-stimulating TV or stereo.

and small amounts of unrefined flaxseed oil. Make sure that you buy organic meats and dairy from pasture-fed cows. You can find omega-3 fatty acids in fish (such as salmon, tuna, trout, and sardines—preferably wild, not farm-raised). Healthy monosaturated fats include peanuts, almonds, pecans, cashews, and avocados—and, of course, my favorite, peanut butter (choose an all-natural and organic brand).

To be sure you are eating healthy fats, first, avoid processed foods that rely on hydrogenated fats—because they are so cheap for manufacturers, they are everywhere in the breads, cereals, energy bars, salad dressings, cake mixes, and peanut butter sold in most grocery stores (you will be much better served at a

Hyperfare Lunch

While breakfast should now be your biggest meal of the day, your lunch is runner-up. Unfortunately, many people either take it lightly, literally—especially those who think that a salad with grilled chicken or a little tuna is all they need—or they get heavy-handed and go to town on a monster-size sandwich, a side of chips or fries, and soda, and then chase it all with a cookie. And people who take a late lunch often overeat because they've given their hunger the chance to rage and end up slowing their metabolism down—a double-whammy that you do not want.

Instead, after having worked out in the morning, or preparing to do so later in the day, lunch is your opportunity to give those muscles the healthy foods they need to recover and perform, and to supply your brain with nutrients to remain alert for the rest of the day. I swear that all-organic, nutrient-dense lunch fare makes or breaks my mental and physical day. Even though I train very hard early each morning, I don't endure the so-called afternoon slump because I feed my body what it's screaming for—a healthy lunch that I make with my own hands.

Of the three main daily meals, your lunch is more likely to be consumed outside of the house. But just as chain restaurants rely on cheap, bad-for-your-waistline-and-overall-health ingredients, typical lunch places can be just as bad, especially if you go to a fast-food joint. Rather than getting a hefty dose of vegetables and complex carbohydrates along with some valuable quality protein—the things your body needs and craves—you usually end up with plain starches and cheap protein (meat and/or cheese) next to a slice of tasteless, usually out-of-season, nutrient-starved lettuce and tomato, and topped with mayo, full of hydrogenated fats. Try to find a lunch place that uses organic ingredients.

You can brown-bag it by preparing your lunch the night before (if you try to slam a sandwich together before you leave for work in the morning, you may either decide to skip it or make an inadequate lunch—and you also add a stressor to your busy morning), and if you have children, you can make their lunch the same way.

The centerpiece of the brown bag lunch is, of course, the sandwich. Use all organic ingredients if you can. Start with two slices of whole-grain fresh bread. Spread some mustard, salsa, olive oil, or vinaigrette lightly on one slice. On the other, use some sliced meat, such as smoked turkey, followed by at least two kinds of vegetables, such as tomatoes, cucumbers, bell peppers, and lettuce (experiment with different kinds, such as watercress and mesclun). Be generous with your sandwich fillings, because you're *not* going to have chips or fries on the side. Instead, couple the meal with a cup of soup, a side salad, some fruit, or smaller amounts of all three.

For a list of recommended lunches, see Appendix A. These lunches can be eaten at home or at work. Sometimes there's nothing better than a hearty fall homemade soup or a cold summer pasta.

SECRET SUMMIT TIP

Isometric Drills

Isometric training is essentially static training in which we apply force to a nonmovable object. I like to call it "hidden strength," because practicing isometric poses builds tremendously strong tendons and helps bind your muscles to the bones—like the chapter title, it links the ladders. Rather than building huge, bloated muscles, it gives you taut and durable muscles.

To me, the epitome of isometric strength was Bruce Lee, who put a heavy emphasis on isometrics and his surprising strength was in part a result of that; he didn't look that strong, but he could simply crush you. Rock climbers also show great isometric strength, being able to support their entire body weight hanging from a finger.

I respect this kind of strength because, again, it's useful in real life—holding a child against your body with your left arm for an entire social gathering, sitting on a stability ball at your desk all day, or balancing on your crampon's front points for an extended period of time while ice climbing. As a result, you will find several isometric moves in the Hyperstrength workouts, such as holding a pull-up halfway up, holding a squat, and staying in a Downward-Facing Dog pose for ten full breaths.

natural foods market). Second, be more selective in the restaurants you choose, as chains are especially notorious for using the cheapest of ingredients to up their profit margin. Third, make your food in the place where you can ensure only the best fats are being used for breakfast, lunch, dinner, and dessert—that is, your very own kitchen.

Hyperstrength, Phase Four: Weeks 7 and 8

Phase Four of Hyperstrength training gives you the opportunity to take the next step in your fitness level. We will focus on cardiovascular and muscular endurance, and whether you're a Trekker, Climber, or Sherpa, you will have longer exercise times, and be working near and above your aerobic ceiling to build lung capacity and threshold. Sherpas will do additional spiked speed training within their cycle drills.

The drills for all levels will now produce higher Hyperfitness Exertion Scale (H.E.S.) numbers, as all levels will perform body-weight, free-weight, and/or

Mike L., Forty-two, Director of Security

"From August 2002 to June 2003, I attended the National Defense University, National War College. Attendees are selected based on their strong leadership skills and the potential they have to be the future leaders of the Department of Defense. From day one, it was made very clear that a key underpinning of a successful leader is a solid physical fitness program. If you are not healthy physically, the odds of being healthy mentally are low. An unhealthy mind directly affects your decision-making process and productivity.

"A morning routine with a solid core of classmates became a daily ritual. As soon as I graduated, I began the search for something to take its place, and Sean Burch's Hyperfitness program did just that, and went way beyond. The program has taken me to levels that I would have never pushed myself to physically because I would not have allowed myself mentally. The Hyperfitness program has significantly expanded my thinking about fitness, and the impact fitness has on every aspect of my day-to-day life.

I am forty-two years old and in the best shape of my life.

"As a federal agent directing security and antiterrorism programs worldwide, the confidence, stamina, and mental fortitude provided by Sean and his program are vital ingredients that enable me to effectively execute our unit's responsibilities in the global war on terrorism. Sean's unique mindset—failure is not an option; give up in here, you will give up out there—is addictive.

"Life is all about setting the goal or expectation and then doing whatever it takes to accomplish or meet it. Great leaders motivate the unit or team toward the stated goal. A great leader gives the unit or team the requisite tools to guarantee success. A great leader leads by example. A great leader never asks anyone to do anything they wouldn't do themselves. Sean pushes himself every day and challenges me to keep up. Sean Burch is a great leader in showing people how a physical fitness routine can grow into a complete lifestyle."

cable exercises. If you are a Sherpa, you should again train for at least one weekend day, choosing a long hike, trail run, recovery, or sport-specific workout. Climbers now have the option to do the same, bumping their training up to six days a week.

Go straight through the 6 drills below, 3 times, with little to no rest between each complete round of exercises. Your body is being introduced to longer exercise times to prepare and challenge you for future level advancements within the program. Stop exercising after 30 to 45 minutes only if your time is absolutely limited, otherwise continue through the drills until you are done.

1. **Stability Ball Individual Dumbbell Chest Press,** 15 reps each arm
2. **Rock Climber,** 4 reps, **to 1 Full Jumping Jack,** 12 reps
3. **Alternating Medicine Ball Push-up** (on your knees if necessary), 10 reps each arm (20 reps total)
4. **Squat to Single Dumbbell Row from Center,** 12 reps each arm
5. **Squat Dumbbell Hammer Curl to Cross-legged Full Jumping Jack,** 15 reps
6. **Squat Two-Hand Medicine Ball Throw** to one bounce, catch and repeat, 20 reps

IE Drill: Go straight through the 3 drills, with little to no rest between them, until you reach 10 minutes (H.E.S. 3–4).

1. **Step Side-to-Side Touches,** 2 sets of 40 reps
2. **Prone Position to Spring,** 30 yards, 5 sets
3. **Frog Jumps,** 3 sets of 20 reps

Hero Pose

Stretch (see pages 58–59)

Stability Ball Individual Dumbbell Chest Press: Get into bench-press position on top of stability ball, with one hand holding a dumbbell, arm straight over chest, and the other stretched out to the side for balance. Switch arms after completing set.

Rock Climber to Full Jumping Jack: Get into push-up position. Keep upper body fixed, then bring right knee to chest and straight again; left knee to chest and straight again; right foot to 3 o'clock and back again; left foot to 9 o'clock and back again. Do in staccato, bouncy rhythm. Then jump both feet to under chest and stand up. Do a jumping jack and repeat.

Alternating Medicine Ball Push-up: Put one hand on the medicine ball and the other hand on the floor for push-ups; switch sides after 10 reps.

Squat to Single Dumbbell Row from Center: Stand on a step or fixed platform and, taking a wide stance, hold on to a dumbbell with one hand between your legs. Squat down and drop the dumbbell lower than the step. Row the dumbbell straight up with one arm as you squat up, keeping your elbow wide.

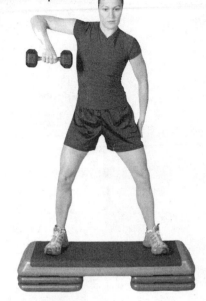

Squat Dumbbell Hammer Curl to Cross-legged Full Jumping Jack: Hold a dumbbell in each hand with palms facing each other at your sides. Squat down and up, then do a hammer curl (thumbs toward your deltoids). Put the weights down, cross your legs, and clap high as you jump.

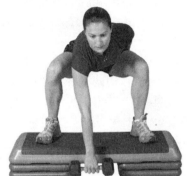

Squat Two-Hand Medicine Ball Throw: Hold the medicine ball in shot-put position with both hands. Squat down and throw the medicine ball up on the way up from the squat as high as you can and/or for distance. Let the ball bounce once, catch, and repeat.

Step Side-to-Side Touches: Standing straight with your left foot on a step with risers or fixed platform placed to your left, push off the left leg and jump over the step. Touch the floor with your left hand while your right foot is on the step. Immediately push off your right foot and jump over the step and touch the floor with your right hand.

Prone Position to Spring: Start in prone position and spring forward, then back to prone position, and repeat.

Frog Jumps: With hands placed on top of head and feet at least shoulder-width apart, slightly angled out, squat down to 90 degrees with your knees going out at the same angle as your toes. Explode forward, jumping like a frog.

Hero Pose: Kneel on floor, keeping legs hip-width apart. Point toes straight back if you can. Relax upper body while stretching quadriceps and tibias anteriors. Hold for 30 seconds.

TREKKER ▲ Weeks 7 and 8 • Tuesday/Thursday

This workout requires access to a treadmill or a trail or grass outdoors (preferably with some hilly areas).

1. Warm up for 5 minutes; jog at 2% incline
2. **Tempo running** for 4 minutes at 3% incline (H.E.S. 2–3)
3. **Climbing with Dumbbells** for 1 minute (H.E.S. 3–4)
4. Do hills until near aerobic threshhold; 4 minute walk or jog at 12% incline (H.E.S. 3)
5. **Incline Push-up** on side of treadmill, 10 reps (H.E.S. 3–4)
6. **Tempo run** near aerobic threshold; 4 minutes at 3% incline (H.E.S. 3)
7. Move side to side (3 strides left to 3 strides right) with dumbbells above your head for 1 minute (H.E.S. 3)
8. Max run above aerobic threshold for 1 minute, at 2% incline (H.E.S. 4)
9. In place, **Squat Jump Touching Wall;** 5 reps slow, 10 reps fast (H.E.S. 3–4)
10. Take a deep breath and say mantra; repeat for 1 minute
11. In place, **Squat Jump Touching Wall;** 5 reps slow, 10 reps fast (H.E.S. 3–4)
12. **Climbing with Dumbbells,** 1 minute (H.E.S. 3–4)
13. Jog for 4 minutes at 2% incline lowering heart rate (H.E.S. 3–1)
14. Jump Rope (with picture of your goal in front of you) 2 min, 30-second rest max, repeat 3 times total (H.E.S. will vary)
15. **Full Smother Crunch,** 15 reps, to Back Extension, 10 reps; repeat 2 times, no rest
16. Hold **Downward Facing Dog Pose** (see page 104) for 4 full breaths

Stretch (see pages 58–59)

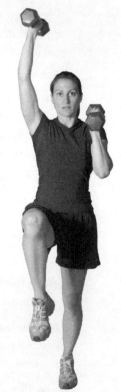

Climbing with Dumbbells: Holding a dumbbell in each hand, with palms facing in and at shoulder height, jog in place and bring your knees as high as possible. At the same time, pump your arms up and down, without locking out your elbows.

Tempo Running: Sustaining a consistent pace near your aerobic threshold.

Incline Push-up on Side of Treadmill: Get into a push-up position, with your hands on the side of the treadmill and feet on the floor. Perform a push-up.

Squat Jump Touching Wall: Facing a wall with your hands over your head, squat until your thighs are almost parallel to the ground and your heels remain on the ground. Explode upward, trying to get maximum height, and touch the wall with the palms of your hands as high up the wall as you can before landing.

Full Smother Crunch: With your back on the stability ball and your feet planted on the floor, bring your head all the way back and cover as much of the ball as you can. Keep your elbows wide and your hands on top of your head. Crunch up.

Back Extension: Lie flat with your face to the ground and stretch your arms out in front of your head. Raise your torso off the ground, keeping your head and arms aligned with your spine while keeping your lower legs on the ground.

CLIMBER ▲▲ Weeks 7 and 8 · Monday/Wednesday/Friday

In the 4 drills that follow, you will perform a set of the first exercise (which is sometimes two exercises combined) and immediately follow with a set of the second exercise. If you cannot complete the reps without stopping, stop and take 1 deep breath, then continue, stopping and taking deep breaths as needed.

1A. **Ring/Strap Push-up with Feet Elevated,** 12 to 15 reps

1B. **Incline Push-up to Dumbbell Jump onto Step,** 10 reps

2A. **Squat Barbell Press Throw Overhead to Catch and Squat Left/Right Knee Up,** 10 reps

2B. **Triangle T to Full Jumping Jack,** 10 reps

3A. **Tabletop Chest Bar Pull-Up to Triceps Push-up,** 10 reps each, 2 times

3B. **Dumbbell Squat, to Jump on Step, to 45-Degree Hammer Curl,** 10 reps

4A. **Medicine Ball Triceps Push-up,** 2 reps, **to Pull-Up with Towel,** 2 reps; perform 10 times

4B. **The "X,"** 15 reps

IE Drill: Repeat the entire IE series for 12 minutes, with a 30-second break in between. Do the series twice. Visualize performing each IE drill perfectly, powerfully. Convince your body mentally that there is so much energy within you that you can complete these exercises without tiring.

1. **V-Sit** (hold for 5 seconds) **to Jump-up;** repeat jumps 5 times in quick succession before returning to V-Sit, 10 reps (H.E.S. 2–3)
2. **Stepleg Cross Jump to Spread-Eagle Step Jump:** Squat jump onto step with risers and cross legs landing on step, 10 reps, to squat jump spread eagle onto step, 10 reps (H.E.S. 3)
3. **Scale the Whale,** up and back on the smooth floor of a basketball court or similar smooth surface, 2 times; mantra yell after each length of court (H.E.S. 3–4)

Hero Pose

Stretch (see pages 58–59)

Ring/Strap Push-up with Feet Elevated: Do ring/strap push-ups with your feet elevated on box or fixed bar, having the rings/handles top at the top of the push-up movement.

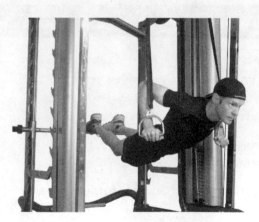 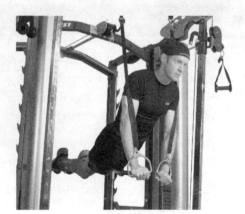

Incline Push-up to Dumbbell Jump onto Step: With each hand on top of a step with risers, get into push-up position. After each push-up, pop your feet under your chest, pick up the dumbbells from the floor with each hand and jump onto the step with the dumbbells by your sides.

Squat Barbell Press Throw Overhead to Catch and Squat Left/Right Knee Up: Squat and press the throw bar (weight added if needed) overhead. Catch, and squat lifting one knee toward your chest as you squat up, squat again, raising the other knee toward your chest as you squat up.

Triangle T to Full Jumping Jack: Start in push-up position with arms straight and feet together. Bring your feet together quickly to the front, back to push-up position, over to the right side, back to push-up position, over to the left side, and back to push-up position. Then bring your feet under your chest and spring up for a full jumping jack.

Tabletop Chest Bar Pull-up to Triceps Push-up: With your feet on a fixed bar or plyometric box, grab rings or straps in each hand and pull your body up as high as possible. Do a triceps push-up on the floor, (performing each with hands on the ground and forming a triangle) immediately after. Complete each rep of both exercises as fast as possible. Two sets complete equals one round.

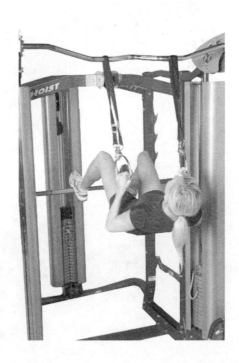

Dumbbell Squat, to Jump on Step, to 45-Degree Hammer Curl: With dumbbells at your sides, squat, having dumbbells touch the floor, and then jump onto a step with at least 3 risers. Follow with a hammer curl on the step, then step down and repeat.

Medicine Ball Triceps Push-up to Pull-up with Towel: Place your hands on the medicine ball and do 2 triceps push-ups. Pop your feet under your chest and stand up. Grab a towel wrapped around the bar and do 2 pull-ups, pulling your head up to the left, and then the right side of the towel.

The "X": Use dumbbells of moderate weight (15 to 30 pounds) and get into a crouched position (all the way down) with dumbbells on the floor on either side of you. Spring out into an X position holding the dumbbells without locking out your elbows. Immediately return to crouched position.

V-Sit to Jump-up: Begin on your back on a step with at least 5 risers and bring both legs and torso off the step to form V. Hold the position for 5 seconds, then roll forward for 5 straight jump-ups, palms touching the floor and jumping as high as possible, bringing arms overhead before returning to V-Sit for next repetition.

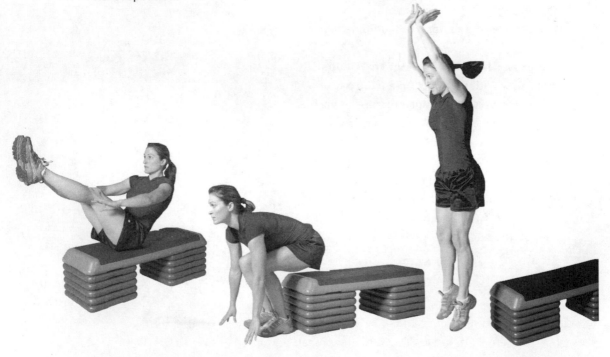

Stepleg Cross Jump to Spread-Eagle Step Jump: With your hands placed on your head, squat jump onto a step with risers, landing on the step with your legs crossed. Repeat 9 times, then squat and perform a spread-eagle jump before landing on the step. Repeat 9 times.

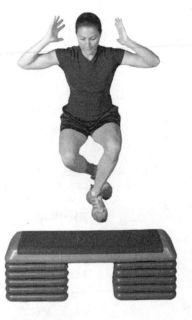

Scale the Whale: With both hands on a towel placed on hard court or smooth surface, get into a set position and run forward.

Hero Pose: Kneel on floor, keeping legs hip-width apart. Point toes straight back if you can. Try to relax upper body while stretching quadriceps and tibias anteriors. Hold for 30 seconds.

CLIMBER ▲▲ Weeks 7 and 8 • Tuesday/Thursday

This workout requires access to a stationary bike.

1. Warm up for 5 minutes on a bike with light resistance and high cadence
2. Cycle drill with medium resistance; alternate out of the saddle to back in the saddle every 4 to 8 beats in tempo for one song (H.E.S. 2–3)
3. Jump back and forth over an obstacle to **Full Jumping Jacks to Split Squats** (sinking your pelvis halfway down); 10 reps each exercise, and repeat 5 times (H.E.S. 3)
4. Cycle sprint with light resistance and high cadence for 1 minute each, with 20-second climbing sprints with heavy resistance in between (go near aerobic threshold); perform 3 times (H.E.S. 3–4)
5. Jump up onto a step with risers or a plyometric box, step down in front, broad jump forward, then run and touch a line 10 yards away; frog jump back to start, jump over step, and repeat; perform 10 times (H.E.S. 3–4)

6. Cycle at medium resistance and do the **Pulse** (triceps push-ups on the handlebars of a bike) throughout, with all-out sprints near aerobic threshold during the chorus for one song (H.E.S. 3)

7. **Bullet Drill** on step or plyo box (loud count of 10 taps) to jump over step, and repeat; perform 11 times (H.E.S. 3)

8. Jump Rope with 2-pound cable; 1 minute on, 15 seconds off; repeat through one song (H.E.S. 3–4)

9. **The Straw:** Cycle at low resistance with consistent cadence for 2–3 minutes

10. **Switch Feet Crunch,** 2 sets of 30 reps

11. Hold **Downward Facing Dog Pose** for 5 full breaths (see page 104)

Stretch (see pages 58–59)

Full Jumping Jacks to Split Squats: Execute a full jumping jack, making sure to clap hands overhead as your legs go out, then clap behind your lower back as your legs come back together. Immediately perform a split squat (bringing one leg out front in a lunge position and bending that leg to 90 degrees) and then jump, switching the other foot forward in midair, and perform another split squat.

Bullet Drill: Quickly bring one foot up to tap step, then the other, then the first back to the ground and other back to the ground. Repeat.

The Straw: Plug your nose and breathe only through a straw. If you become dizzy, immediately remove straw and breathe normally.

Switch Feet Crunch: Lie on the ground with legs extended and one foot stacked on top of the other off the ground. Crunch, lifting your shoulder blades off the floor and raising your chest toward the ceiling, and switch feet as you crunch.

CLIMBER ▲▲ Weeks 7 and 8 • Saturday (Optional)

Choose a Recovery Workout provided for you in Appendix D, a recovery workout of your own creation, or a sport-specific recovery workout.

In the following 3 intense drills, you perform a set of the first exercise (which is sometimes two moves combined), immediately followed by a set of the second exercise, and then a third exercise. Take a few deep breaths, then repeat each drill twice more. After the 3 sets of each drill, rest for at least 2 minutes (or the time it takes to organize equipment for the next drill) before moving to the next one.

1A. **Jump Push-up Holding Dumbbells,** 15 reps
1B. **Upside-Down Pull-up,** 10 reps
1C. **Bosu One-Leg Crunch** (switch legs every 5 reps), 20 reps

2A. **Wide Push-up, to Triceps Push-up with Feet in Rings/Straps** (to exhausted state), **to Cycle Spin and Dumbbell Fly** at same time, 10 times
2B. **Knee High Underneath Claps,** 4 reps, to **Squat Jump Daffies,** 3 reps; 10 times
2C. **Push-up Hold with Straps, to Spread Eagle, to V,** 20 reps

3A. **Rings/Straps Skullcrusher to Fly,** 12 reps
3B. **Pterodactyl,** 5 reps, **to Donkey Kick, to Jump up and Legs out Clap;** 15 reps
3C. **Squat Single-Arm Dumbbell/Kettlebell Diagonals on One Leg,** 12 reps each arm

IE Drill 1: After both of the IE drills, do a 1-minute visualization and mantra yells. Repeat the series 2 more times (H.E.S. 3–4).

  1. **Beached Whale,** 10 reps each side (20 reps total)
  2. **Evolution of Frog Jump 5–9;** 20 yards up and back, 2 reps each variation

IE Drill 2: (H.E.S. 4)

  1. Jump Rope with a 3-pound cable as fast as possible to exhausted state; stop, take 2 deep breaths, and repeat 4 times more

Downward Facing Dog Pose, hold for 10 full breaths

Stretch (see pages 58–59)

Jump Push-up Holding Dumbbells: With a dumbbell in each hand, do a push-up, lifting the dumbbells off the floor as you push up.

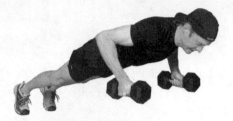

Upside-Down Pull-up: Grab the bar and place your body in an upside-down position with your legs bent and knees directly in front of your face. Extend your legs straight up as you pull up.

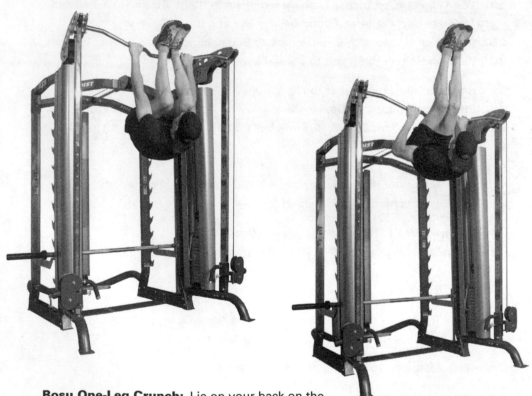

Bosu One-Leg Crunch: Lie on your back on the Bosu with one leg off the ground and the other bent at 90 degrees supporting. Crunch up while bringing the raised knee to your chest. Use a 5-second count on the way back down.

Wide Push-up, to Triceps Push-up with Feet in Rings/Straps, to Cycle Spin and Dumbbell Fly: Secure your feet in rings or straps and get into push-up position. Complete a set of wide-stance push-ups and then pop your hands next to each other for triceps push-ups (with each triceps push-up done with hands on the ground forming a triangle). Next, immediately lie on your back on the floor for Cycle Spin (spin your legs in the air as if cycling) while doing Dumbbell Flys at same time.

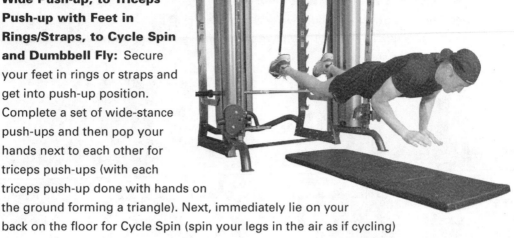

Dumbbell Fly: Lie on your back holding a dumbbell in each hand, with your arms straight out at your sides and slightly bent. While performing cycle spins (spin your legs in the air as if cycling), bring the dumbbells together above your head.

Knee High Underneath Claps to Squat Jump Daffies: Run in place, bringing your knees to your chest and clapping your hands underneath each stride, for 4 strides, then squat down with palms touching the ground and jump up while one leg goes in front and the other in back.

Push-up Hold with Straps, to Spread Eagle, to V: Put each foot in a strap, get into push-up position with arms straight, and hold for 1 second. Spread your legs apart and hold for 1 second. Then close your legs as you raise your glutes in the air as high as possible, and hold for 1 second.

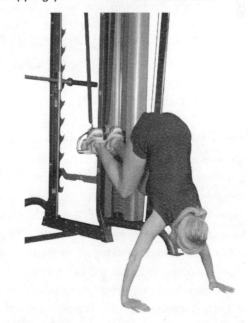

Rings/Straps Skullcrusher to Fly: Hold a ring or strap in each hand and get into incline push-up position, with extended arms. Do a triceps press-down until the rings/straps touch your forehead and then extend your arms again. Then fly both rings/straps out to the sides.

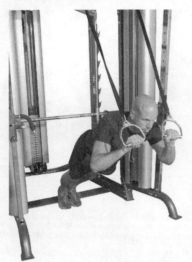 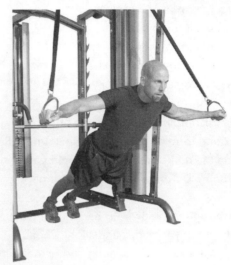

Pterodactyl, to Donkey Kick, to Jump up and Legs out Clap: From standing position, go to push-up position with your feet together. Bring your feet together under you, then back, then under you. Repeat 5 times. Then, on your next kickback, kick both legs straight out behind you in the air. Then jump up and kick your legs apart out to the side while clapping your hands in front of you, then bring your legs together and as you land clap your hands behind you.

Squat Single-Arm Dumbbell/Kettlebell Diagonals on One Leg: Balance on your left leg and bend your right leg at 90 degrees, while you hold a dumbbell or kettlebell in your right hand. Squat down on your left leg, while bringing the kettlebell as far from the outside left leg as possible. Rise from the squat, bringing the kettlebell diagonally across your body and over your right shoulder. Switch sides after completing the set.

Beached Whale: Jump over a step with at least 4 risers or a plyo box, then do 1 rollover sideways and jump straight up with your hands above your head. Roll back, side jump over the step, roll over, and jump straight up with your hands above your head. Repeat.

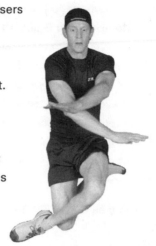

Evolution of Frog Jump 5–9: First, squat jump forward, placing your palms on the floor; second, squat jump spread-eagle to palms touching the floor; third, squat jump daffy (scissorslike position) to palms touching the floor; fourth, squat jump spread-eagle to palms touching the floor to squat jump daffy to palms touching the floor; last, squat jump legs and arms cross to palms touch the floor.

SHERPA ▲▲▲ Weeks 7 and 8 · Tuesday/Thursday

You'll need a stationary bike for these exercises. Pick songs with powerful, steady beats throughout the entire session.

1. Warm up for 5 minutes at a moderate pace at 75 rpm (H.E.S. 1–2)
2. Cycle at medium-light resistance and do the **Pump Cross** (bend your arms, push off the handlebars with your hands, and cross your arms in front of you) for one song. During the chorus of the song, do sprints, staying off the seat. (Example of a song to use: Rage Against the Machine's "The Ghost of Tom Joad") (H.E.S. 2–3)
3. **The HB,** 15 yards up and back, 5 times (H.E.S. 3)
4. Cycle at medium resistance and bend forward to do triceps push-ups on the handlebars of the bike throughout one song, with all-out seated sprints during the chorus (H.E.S. 3)
5. Get off the bike and **Barbell Squat Jump Forward** 111 times (H.E.S. 3)
6. Cycle at steady medium to high resistance for 1 song, out of the saddle. Then sing 2 songs out loud while keeping an aerobic pace from seated to out of saddle climbing (H.E.S. 3–4)
7. **The HB,** 15 yards up and back, 5 times (H.E.S. 3)
8. Cycle sprint with low resistance, at least 110 rpm for 1 song (H.E.S. 3–4)
9. **Barbell Squat Jump Forward,** 111 times (H.E.S. 3–4)

10. 2 minute deep breaths (H.E.S. to 1)
11. **Medicine Ball Stairwell Drill;** repeat mantras during the drill, 10 minutes (alternative if no stairwell: repeat #6) (H.E.S. 3)
12. **Weighted Runs,** on basketball court or outside grass; 3 times up and back for each, for 20 yards each exercise (H.E.S. 3–4)
13. **Medicine Ball Stairwell Drill;** repeat mantras during the drill, 10 minutes (alternative if no stairwell: repeat #6) (H.E.S. 3)
14. **Weighted Runs,** on basketball court or outside grass; 3 times up and back for each, for 20 yards each exercise (H.E.S. 3–4)
15. **Hero Pose**

Stretch (see pages 58–59)

The HB: Squat jump forward, then have your knees and palms touch the ground. Repeat.

Barbell Squat Jump Forward: Place a 45-pound barbell behind your neck and jump forward, focusing on short, powerful, sharp exhalations with each breath, forcing your lungs to work harder. If you feel dizzy, stop, catch your breath, and then continue.

Medicine Ball Stairwell Drill: Holding 2 medicine balls of different weights, first do knee-highs up the stairs and jog down; next, skip a step going up and jog down; last, skip 2 steps going up and jog down.

Weighted Runs: For each version, go down and back holding a dumbbell or kettlebell. First, hold the dumbbell in one hand; next, rickshaw (hold the dumbbell behind you at glute level); next, hold the dumbbell with both hands out in front; next, hold the dumbbell above your head; last, hold the dumbbell in one hand while running backward.

Hero Pose: Kneel on floor, keeping legs hip-width apart. Point toes straight back if you can. Try to relax upper body while stretching quadriceps and tibias anteriors. Hold for 30 seconds.

SHERPA ▲▲▲ Weeks 7 and 8 · Saturday

Choose a Recovery Workout provided for you in Appendix D, a long hike or trail run, a recovery workout of your own creation, or a sport-specific recovery workout.

Chapter 7

PERSEVERING IN THE DEATH ZONE

Weeks 9 and 10

Afterwards having climbed most of
the intimidating Lhotse Face on my journey up Everest, I dropped into my tent
at Camp 3, which was, literally, fixed to narrow ledges of the steep ice wall. By
far the most dangerous camp on the climb, it is vulnerable to unpredictable
weather and avalanches. Because of this, many Sherpas opt not to stay at this
camp and are strong enough to make it to the South Col in one long day from
Camp 2. We lowlanders, however, struggle mightily with the altitude, and need
the rest.

Exhausted, I took in as many calories as I could keep down, eating all-
natural breakfast cookies and various soups—at this altitude, your resting heart
rate is so high that you lose weight no matter how much food you devour—and
even the energy gels were becoming difficult to stomach. I tried to sleep while
the walls of my tent shook from the relentless wind. I knew that I had just overcome one the biggest physical challenges of my life, but my excitement was tem-
pered. After spending two days of rest at Camp 3 because of poor weather
conditions, I was headed to Camp 4 on the South Col, which at 26,300 feet is
known as "the death zone"—and my body seemed to know it already.

I was starting to show the beginning signs of altitude sickness. Like seasickness, it sounds innocuous until you get it. Even at Base Camp, the amount of available oxygen was just half of that at sea level. By the time I reached Camp 4, it would plummet to a third. As a result, from Camp 3 onward, 90 percent of Western climbers use bottled oxygen. The now standard practice of the big oxygen assist, however, offers no guarantees for a successful summit, as one's judgment and coordination can still deteriorate rapidly, while severe fatigue takes over your body and pounding headaches, vomiting, and diarrhea take their toll.

During my climb to Camp 4, those wretched bodily symptoms were already showing up, probably prematurely invited by my decision not to use any bottled oxygen. Being a climbing purist, my intention all along was never to take in supplementary oxygen unless I really felt I was in danger of dying.

I remained confident of my ability to keep death at bay, principally because of the rigorous mental and physical training I'd undergone before my journey. What I couldn't stave off, however, was the headache knocking inside my head, the primary symptom of altitude sickness. The headache stayed with me all the while I tried to fight through my physical exhaustion. Because of the lack of oxygen, at times I moved no faster than a toddler first learning to walk. I gave up trying to ingest any food, as I just couldn't keep it down and my appetite was missing in action. Finally, by day's end, I dragged my body up to Camp 4 at the South Col.

South Col essentially functions as a mountain pass to Everest's summit. While it's a celebrated and cherished place to reach, in reality it's a lonely, desolate, frozen, windswept, and rock-ridden area. Jet streams are constant, with storm winds coming up on you rapidly. Because of these winds, the picturesque Everest snow—which also functions as valuable insulation around your tent—is scarce.

By the time I reached the South Col, I hadn't eaten in more than twelve hours—and I'd had barely any water. It was almost like having food poisoning, as my nausea and periodic dizziness came in waves. Each breath became labored, as my throat seemed clogged with blood that had turned into molasses.

I began to feel increasingly confused as I started to exhibit more severe signs of altitude sickness. Most of the climbers who die up here essentially have their minds shut down on them just before their bodies do, as extreme symptoms include psychosis, hallucinations, and confusion.

I had to distinguish between what was normal at this altitude and what could spell the end. The threat of frostbite and hypothermia is ever-present, so I made sure to always keep moving in some way, and especially to keep moving my toes and fingers. In the death zone, nonessential body functions are temporarily shut down, as sleeping becomes nearly impossible and digesting food *is* impossible. Staying longer than two or three days in the death zone makes your body deteriorate rapidly, until you lose consciousness and die. I came across several reminders of such a grim fate, and saw dead climbers still clad in their colorful climbing apparel. They could have died yesterday or many years ago because, as a result of the extreme cold, almost no decomposition occurs above Camp 4. Of course, I never looked too carefully.

Making Your Mark

In the ninth and tenth weeks, you may start to feel as though you're entering the death zone. But you can push through and utilize this program to transform your life, as I did. So why enter an area called the death zone? Because, simply, if you complete each of these workouts, then there's nothing else in life that you can't do.

If you stick with the program in these weeks, you'll experience something beyond the endorphin-fueled "runner's high"; you'll get a deeper sense of accomplishment. If that sounds like an exaggeration, wait until it hits you and you realize that you have control over your destiny, something few people ever realize. You, perhaps for the first time in your life, have become powerful and capable of great, unimaginable things.

The prudent thing for me to have done would have been to turn around in the death zone after my failed first evening summit attempt. I'd already spent almost twenty-four hours there, and I knew that another evening ascent and descent would put me in grave physical danger. On Everest, a climber who uses up all his energy to get to the summit likely perishes on the descent. Going to the limit in other extreme adventures, like a triathlon or marathon, might mean you don't finish the race, but you still live to race another day. But that same all-out performance in which you might come up short will only get you killed on Everest.

I knew that my chance of succeeding on back-to-back summit day attempts from the South Col was very unlikely, and I was aware that my body was slowly dying from the lack of oxygen. Plus high winds made any attempt to climb higher foolish. The situation looked bleak, as four years of planning and tens of thousands of dollars spent on organization, equipment, and training were slipping away. I sank into a depression, knowing now that the summit, only a few thousand feet away, was most likely out of reach.

My only course was to sleep. That early morning, I tossed and turned, struggling to stay warm and positive. By midday, my inner fortitude had returned. It dawned on me that this was the biggest moment in my life up until that point. Eager to make the most of my situation, I decided to jump rope at 26,181 feet, which broke my old world record.

Most important, I decided that I'd try to make a second push for the summit that evening, but only if the weather cooperated. Often the weather was favorable during the dark hours. If either the mountain or Mother Nature didn't give the opportunity, I decided I could live with it. I was certain that everything I'd worked so hard for and learned along the way had made me a better person. Whether or not I got to the summit wouldn't change that. If I had to turn around, I'd have no regrets.

You Can Either Give in to the World, or Change It

Conquering the "quit factor" and remaining positive amid trying circumstances is how you attain the life experience you want. Your desire, preparation, and spirit will be tested many times, especially when you're tired, dejected, or overwhelmed. Will you persevere in spite of the doubts and fatigue?

BODY CHECK

Weeks 9 and 10

As you know, in each week of the program there are at least two separate workouts. I designed it that way not only to keep everything fresh and fun, but also because the Monday/Wednesday/Friday workout periodically pushes you into the anaerobic zone (high intensity) while the Tuesday/Thursday (and sometimes Saturday, depending on your level) hovers more in your aerobic zones (moderate intensity).

I've done this because it's not wise to train in either of the zones on consecutive days, because you wouldn't be giving your body enough time to recover from each mode of training, which can cause symptoms of overtraining. Signs of overtraining include excessive muscle soreness that doesn't go away, joint aches, lack of energy, drop in performance, insomnia, headaches, insatiable thirst, and lower resistance to common illnesses.

Working in your anaerobic zone, your body will produce lactic acid—indicators include rapid breathing, a burning sensation in your muscles, and an increase in your heart rate. It is very difficult to maintain a period of intense anaerobic activity (H.E.S. Sector 4 HyperMax; see Appendix E) for more than thirty seconds to two minutes before having to slow down, but you can improve your lactate threshold, which is your body's ability to tolerate lactic acid. As your threshold improves, so do your performance levels. (See page 39 for more on lactic acid.)

This type of high-intensity training will churn out the endorphins, a.k.a. the "runner's high," after a set period of time. However, don't come to depend upon this high, because steady-state workouts (the workouts in which you don't fluctuate too much within the aerobic zone) and active rest days are just as essential to steadily improving your fitness level without overdoing it.

Make sure you're adequately hydrated and eating your daily Hyperfare meals (protein, clean carbs, and good fats) during the day, and start each workout with some solid nutrition "on board." For example, if you're working out for over an hour, take in some calories and perhaps a low-calorie electrolyte drink.

At this point in the program, you're way stronger than you used to be, and more efficient at doing the exercises more consecutively without rest. By continuing to access your hy-ki, facing any fears that arise, and uniting your entire being to take on all challenges, you can taste success. The short-term goals are more tangible than ever before, and hopefully you're also more resolute and ready for your own long-term Inner Everest goal.

To gauge your progress as well as what still may hold you back from true success, read through the following self-evaluation questions and jot down your answers in your Hyperfitness journal. They will be very useful later on.

- Do you spend time asking yourself "What if?" questions?
- Are you quitting your workouts before they're finished, or do you stick it out for entire sessions?
- Do you feel like quitting the program right now because the effort feels like it's too much for you?
- Do you see obstacles as dreaded barriers that may throw you off course, or are they hurdles that you relish overcoming?
- Do you look only for guarantees in most everyday situations?
- Do you have a tendency to fail at projects if your goals are not reached quickly?

Answering these questions honestly will show your progress and highlight what you need to work on. Having humility and keeping an open mind in front of your upcoming tasks, no matter how large, will help eliminate frustration and keep your energy positive and proactive. If things have to go well in the beginning or middle of your march toward your goals, then you're really not committed to your cause; if you rely on guarantees along the way, then you're not putting much at risk.

I don't want to see you fall into comfort zones and land well below your full potential. If I had stayed in my comfort zone and away from risk during my Everest climb, I'd have turned around at Base Camp. It still would have been a good experience, but I would have known that it was far short of what I was really capable of.

Numerous times in your life, you've probably already been presented with the "quit factor." A relationship turns rocky, a job venture becomes tricky, a sport gets you injured—so you quit. It's easy, because all you have to do is stop: stop calling your mate back, stop showing up at work, stop training for your sport. You're told, "It wasn't meant to be." "Hey, it's okay. No big deal." "I told you you were insane to start playing soccer again." Today's society tells you how to be a compliant, easygoing loser.

Because this is life, not every task you set out to do works out like you had planned and at times you may be temped to give up. Many people start an exercise program and give up after a few months, because they tell themselves (or others tell them) it's too hard, they don't have enough time, or the program just doesn't work for them. You must always stay positive and see the task through, all the way to its conclusion. If, for example, you kept to that fitness program faithfully for six months and you stopped seeing results, maybe you were right to think it's not for you. But that doesn't mean that your search to become more fit and strong suddenly screeches to a halt; rather, you just have to find something better (Hyperfitness, of course). Otherwise, whether it's true or not, it just looks like you were looking for an excuse to quit.

Even in the cases where you don't reach the specific target you had set, by not giving up, you'll actually end up coming much closer to your goal than you would have otherwise. Plus you've gained some valuable knowledge that you can use elsewhere, such as tackling your very next, and perhaps related, goal. Transferring your energy to the new goal, in addition to using this know-how, will give you a head start.

Even so-called "failures" who tried are happier than those who never did. Do you want merely to sit on the porch when you're old, daydreaming about "what if I'd done that, or maybe this"? I say, stick out your neck into the blustery wind of chance—that is where you can reach harmony of yourself with the earth, and where achievement and contentment dwell.

When I go on an expedition or take on any type of project, I never ponder the question, "What if I fail?" When you are on your path toward achieving your dream goals, such a self-defeating question should never enter your mind. Personally, I have "lost" many times, but I never equate a loss with failing because I always value it as a learning experience. When dealing with something as vital as your dream goals, be patient and realize that many developments take time. Believe me, this is something that I often have to remind myself of! For example, my energy levels are usually higher, and I may see the goal a bit differently than others I work with—so I try to be patient with them, while at the same time operate as a motivating force.

To embolden and energize you for the final stages of the climb toward your short-term goal, you must commit to superhuman effort. Accumulate the small wins along the way, and slap yourself on the back for them—the workouts completed, the days that you eat only healthy foods, the progress you make toward your long-term goals, the positive attitude that you bring to everything. Hopefully you have others in your life that will also give you that back slap, supporting and encouraging you along the way, just as you do the same for them. Meanwhile, stay away as best as you can from the mental hurdles you may have faced in the past, such as losing your temper, getting depressed, showing impatience, feeling sorry for yourself, or failing to have a sense of humor about it all. I want you to take yourself and your goals very seriously, but not so seriously that you forget to smile and laugh along the way, especially when the going gets a little rough. Many people who've done well in sports and other life pursuits credit their sense of humor, and not taking themselves too seriously, for allowing them the freedom to succeed.

Whatever you do, make every effort never to abandon your good intentions, for yourself and others. Stay engaged each step of the way. This program, through mental, physical, and nutritional conditioning, builds an unprecedented level of confidence and focus so you can see those intentions through.

Keeping Your Fire Stoked: Getting a HyperMetabolism

A lot of people who struggle with their weight blame their metabolism. Every so often, someone will tell me, "You're so lucky that you have such a fast metabolism! You couldn't do what you've done if you had mine." Because this is usually meant as a kind of compliment (though it never feels like one), it actually irritates me on many levels. Although genetics plays a role (as can an underactive thyroid gland or imbalanced hormone levels), we can directly affect the speed of our metabolism. Do you think my fast metabolism and lean physique has something to do with my practice of exercising six or more days a week, along with eating proper amounts of good nutrition at regular intervals? I'd answer with a resounding "yes."

The most common mistake of those with a "slow metabolism" is infrequent eating, or the no-breakfast, small-lunch, and big-dinner routine. This kind of pattern is actually making the body's metabolism slow down, even if it was boosted by exercise, because it's not receiving food in the morning after eight to ten hours going without anything. The message of "starving!" is sent and your survival mechanism kicks in, and as a result your metabolism slows down. When you finally do introduce some calories around lunchtime, the body is more likely to turn them into fat in order to preserve itself for future signals of starvation.

We burn through our calories in three major ways: our resting metabolic rate (RMR), the thermic effect of food (TEF), and our energy expenditure (EE). Our RMR represents the number of calories we burn at rest, and it accounts for about 60 to 75 percent of our total daily calorie expenditure. The TEF involves the simple practice of eating food, especially the digestion, absorption, and storage of food within our bodies; it makes up about 5 to 10 percent of the total calories we burn each day.

The last component is the component that is most in your control: exercise! It can account for 20 to 30 percent of your total daily calorie expenditure. That's huge, of course. Your EE is not just your workout, but also the other physical activities that do add up, as in calories burnt—having a job that requires physical activity, walking or cycling to the market rather than driving, taking the stairs rather than the elevator, standing and moving around the kitchen for an hour while cooking a meal, playing with your child in the yard for half an hour, and so on.

With the Hyperstrength workouts, your EE gets the biggest increase possible in the workout department. The fact that you are frequently working out during the week—and at high intensities for significant durations—means that your metabolism is receiving the maximum boost from exercise. Studies demonstrate that while cardiovascular-only exercise (such as a three-mile jog or a thirty-minute walk on the treadmill) gives you approximately a two-hour metabolic boost, mixing strength training into each workout (which every Hyperstrength session does) raises your metabolism for a full forty-eight hours. Increasing the amount of muscle in your body through regular weight training can boost your

RMR by 15 percent. This is because muscle is metabolically active and burns more calories than other body tissue, even when you're not moving. For every extra pound of muscle you put on, your body uses about 50 extra calories a day. Again, you can see how exercise can make the difference between having what is conventionally referred to as a "fast" or "slow" metabolism.

Because your metabolism, if left undisturbed by exercise and other variables, can decline by 1 percent each year after the age of 30, it's important that you do whatever you can in your power to keep it revved up.

Rather than recommend the six or seven mini-meal approach, I'm old-school in this one department: the best eating schedule for your metabolism is three regular meals, plus two to three small snacks per day (80–150 calories), depending upon your exercise level. And remember, different types of foods change how many calories are burnt after you've eaten them. For every 100 calories of fat you eat, your body uses up five; for 100 calories of complex, clean carbohydrates you take in, your body burns 10 calories; and for every 100 calories of protein ingested, your body torches 20 to 30 calories.

The Hyperfare eating plan works perfectly for your metabolism because it has ample quantities of healthy protein and carbohydrates, along with a moderate amount of good fat. Those fanatical about their weight go on the Catch-22 Plan, as they suddenly try to exercise a lot *and* eat much less. Not only do fewer calories mean their workouts will end prematurely but also their metabolism will have no choice but to slow down; then whatever exercise they do get in won't show much benefit.

Increasing your metabolism is a fancy way of saying 'stoking your furnace,' because that's how your metabolism functions in the body. As we've discussed, exercise and food creates extra heat in the body, on top of our resting metabolic rate and the heat it generates. Combining the two, such as taking a slow stroll after dinner, aids in digestion and heats up that metabolism a little more.

Caffeine, too, creates heat and can provide that extra kick you need for your workout, but I caution you to not overuse it. Personally, I recommend going with tea, which isn't as high in caffeine as coffee and is a far cry from thermogenic drinks. Instead, I love organic yerba mate tea, which is grown in the rain

Hyperfare Dinner

Eating quality proteins, low-glycemic carbohydrates, and good fats in the evening promotes muscle recovery during your sleep, and after your Hyperstrength workout each day, a recovery meal is exactly what the doctor will have ordered.

Ideally, this meal you should be cooked at home, where you can control everything that goes on your plate. You've taken the time to train properly, so spend some time in your kitchen as well. Many great meals can be made in 20 to 45 minutes, and your body (as well as any other people in your household) will thank you for it. In my world, sitting around the dinner table with my loved ones, talking about life, and eating the delicious food that my wife or I have just prepared is as good as it gets.

For ideas about what to cook, see Appendix A. The best of Hyperfare meals begin with great ingredients, of course, like vegetables, meats, herbs, and spices from your farmers' market, CSA (community-supported agriculture), or natural foods store. If these ingredients are high quality, locally grown, organic, and seasonal—try to hit on all four elements whenever possible—you'll find it's actually hard to screw up a meal.

Last, perhaps contrary to what you're used to, dinner should be the smallest meal of the day, so watch your portions. And don't eat within two hours of bedtime, or you'll shortchange your metabolism, your digestion may be affected, and it may be harder to fall asleep.

forest, and I drink it daily. It contains some caffeine, along with catechins—which help move fat molecules through the body faster than other liquids—and tons of antioxidants, which help prevent the buildup of free radicals from my hard training. Green tea also delivers both caffeine and antioxidants.

Last, give spicy foods a go. Studies have demonstrated that your metabolic rate can be increased by up to 50 percent for up to three hours after a spicy meal. I love all kinds of spicy food, whether Thai, Mexican, American, or Japanese. And when the meal isn't so spicy, I'll douse the plate with red pepper flakes.

Hyperstrength, Phase Four: Weeks 9 and 10

As you begin the ninth week of the Hyperstrength program, you will work on tandem muscular and cardiovascular exercising. In essence, you will use all of your major muscle groups jointly in every exercise drill to build a higher level of athleticism. Trekkers and Climbers will use dumbbell weights and/or cable

George C., Forty-two, U.S. Government Bureau Chief

"I've been training with Sean for nine years. When I started in 1998, I was just looking for self-defense instruction to protect my family and me. Little did I know that Sean's expertise would give me so much more.

"Thanks to Sean, I was able to blend confidence, focus, and discipline into a successful career track. In 1998, despite having worked in the U.S. government for nine years, I was still a junior-grade employee, having had only two promotions with no clear vision of how I was going to achieve my goals. Training with Sean—learning from Sean—not only built my physical conditioning and self-defense skills, but also instilled confidence and discipline that helped me dramatically accelerate my career. I went from two promotions in nine years pre-Sean to six promotions in nine years post-Sean. The number of awards I received tripled after I started working with Sean. I rose from a run-of-the-mill analyst with no supervisory role to the deputy chief of a sixty-five-person group, the latter at a grade lower than most people will even be considered for the position. Sure, I worked hard for these achievements, but I had worked hard before 1998, too. You can bang as hard as you want to to try to open a door, but a key is so much easier.

"Training with Sean melded the key for me, and I've benefited greatly. I'm still learning from every session with Sean; the sessions are critical to my job satisfaction and focus. In addition to being a world-class instructor, Sean is an extraordinary man. Despite his world-record accomplishments, Sean focuses more on other people—his family, his friends, and his students—than he does on himself. It was this blend of accomplishment and compassion—and earthshaking passion, let me tell you—that drove me up a 4,500-foot mountain during a recent hike. I had never hiked a mountain this high, and even though it was minuscule by Sean's standards, it was my Everest (as Sean himself pointed out to me). It was far more difficult than I could have imagined. Forget wooded, grassy paths—this was a boulder-strewn, stone-laden maze you could just barely call a path. Going up was tough; struggling down was tougher. I was getting schooled, and I didn't like it. However, every time I felt as if I couldn't make it up the mountain, every time I felt as if my burning quads were going to give way down the mountain, I heard Sean's voice in my head: "Breathe, focus, brother. Are you going to let this mountain beat you? How bad do you want it?" The truth was, I wanted it bad. The mountain tempted me, taunted me, but I never could have met the challenge without Sean. His teachings—both physical and mental—again provided me with the key.

"Take it from me: you've never really seen energy and inspiration unless you know, have met, or read the words of Sean Burch. Take a read; it'll do you good—for a lifetime."

exercises for core building, while Sherpas will continue to use novel Hyperstrength exercises.

All levels will see improved muscular strength, with minimal to no rest between sets to increase muscular and cardiovascular endurance. Conditioning

Steve P., Forty-one, Construction Director

"Sean Burch has made a dramatic improvement in my life over the five months that I have known him. My goals were simple: improve my fitness so that I could play with my children, and improve my golf and tennis games. I had limited fitness and several previous sports injuries, which I thought were limiting what I could achieve.

"The Hyperfitness program that he put me on was the most physically challenging I have experienced, and one of his mantras, 'put in the effort, and you will get the results,' was true when I started and is still true today.

"His program made me 'functional,' meaning I am now capable of participating in a wide variety of sports, including biking, tennis, running, volleyball, soccer, and so on.

"A solid benefit of his Hyperfitness training is the mental side of fitness. He brings a unique intensity and focus to fitness that strips away the distractions and the 'can't-do's' that can easily impair the effectiveness of a program.

"Now I am challenged with seeking out new fitness goals, since I have achieved and exceeded the fitness goals I had five months ago, and have recently set a new personal best in golf and ridden my bike four times farther than I had previously."

will consist of hill training for anaerobic development and tempo training for aerobic endurance. Climbers and Sherpas will continue IE drills that stress balance and elevated aerobic endurance, while Trekkers' IE drills will focus on maximizing their anaerobic potential while building their real-life strength.

Meanwhile, the weekend exercise regimen for Climbers is now mandatory to help them establish body awareness and promote active recovery. As the program enters its final stages, Climbers and Sherpas are training their bodies to be able to exercise daily without reservation.

TREKKER ▲ Weeks 9 and 10 • Monday/Wednesday/Friday

Go straight through the 6 drills below, 3 times, with little to no rest between each complete round of exercises. Your body is being introduced to longer exercise times to prepare and challenge you for future level advancements and longer workouts within the program. Do your best to complete the entire session each day.

1. **Dumbbell Squat, to Overhead Press, to Calf Raise,** 14 reps
2. **Decline Push-ups with Feet on Stability Ball,** 45 seconds
3. **Squat Jump Circles with Medicine Ball,** 10 reps clockwise, 10 reps counterclockwise
4. **Medicine Ball Crunch Throw and Catch on Stability Ball,** 15 reps
5. **Dumbbell One-Arm Squat to Diagonal Press,** 12 reps each arm
6. **Medicine Ball Triceps Push-up,** max out, **to** 5 reps **Jump Squats,** 6 reps

IE Drill: Use steps with risers, a plyometrics box, or a bench for these 3 drills. Go straight through all 3, with little to no rest between them, and repeat once more. Complete the series 2 times total (H.E.S. 3–4).

1. **Squat Jump, to Incline Push-up, to Jumping Jack,** 10 reps
2. **Straddle Step Jump with Dumbbells,** 10 reps
3. **Toe Taps,** 6 reps, **to Jump-overs,** 10 reps

Standing Waist Roll, 1 minute

Stretch (see pages 58–59)

Dumbbell Squat, to Overhead Press, to Calf Raise: Holding a dumbbell in each hand, squat down until the dumbbells reach the floor then bring them up to shoulder level on your way up. Press overhead, palms facing in, while raising up on your calves.

Decline Push-ups with Feet on Stability Ball: Position your hands in push-up position and put the top of your feet on top of the stability ball. Extend your legs out so that from your head to your ankles your body forms a straight line, and perform push-ups. If you cannot complete the full time before stopping, bend to your knees and then continue.

Squat Jump Circles with Medicine Ball: With the medicine ball held to your chest, squat jump upward and make full turns with the medicine ball.

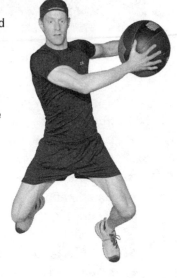

Medicine Ball Crunch Throw and Catch on Stability Ball: Hold the medicine ball overhead while crunching on the stability ball. On the way up, throw the ball into the air. Catch overhead, and return to a crunch.

Dumbbell One-Arm Squat to Diagonal Press: Stand with your right hand holding a dumbbell at your side. Squat down and bring the dumbbell to the side of your inner left foot. Squat up and bring the weight all the way overhead and over your right shoulder. Switch sides after doing a set.

Medicine Ball Triceps Push-up to Jump Squats: With hands on a medicine ball and forming a triangle, do a triceps push-up. Then pop feet under chest and jump up off the ground as high as possible.

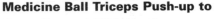

Squat Jump, to Incline Push-up, to Jumping Jack: Jump onto a platform, step back down, then place your hands out to push-up position on the platform and do an incline push-up. Next, bring your legs under your chest, come up, and do full jumping jack.

Straddle Step Jump with Dumbbells: Straddle a step with your legs, and then squat down and jump, holding dumbbells. Switch which foot lands first when stepping down after each jump.

Toe Taps to Jump-overs: Alternating your feet, tap the top of a step with at least 4 risers as quickly as you can. Next, place one leg on the platform, push off that leg, and jump over the platform. Repeat on the other side.

Standing Waist Roll: Place your hands on your hips, keeping your back straight, and roll your upper body in hula hoop–like circle.

TREKKER ▲ Weeks 9 and 10 • Tuesday/Thursday

This workout ("The 5s") requires access to a treadmill, wooden court surface, and/or outside grass (H.E.S. 2–4).

1. Dumbbells by your side, run forward 30 yards; run back with dumbbells in front of your chest (lock out your arms); repeat for 5 minutes
2. **Dumbbell Split Squat Jumps Forward** (knees go halfway down) 30 yards; run back with dumbbells in front of your chest; repeat for 5 minutes.
3. **Frog Jump** forward with dumbbells between your legs 30 yards; run back with dumbbells in front of your chest; repeat for 5 minutes.
4. Dumbbells above your head running forward 30 yards; run back with dumbbells in front of your chest; repeat for 5 minutes.
5. 15% incline jog for 5 minutes.
6. 5 **Dumbbell Push-ups,** to 5 **Squat Jumps** in place, to 5 **Dumbbell Push-ups** to 5 **Dumbbell Squat Jumps;** repeat 5 times total.
7. 5% incline run for 5 minutes.
8. 5 **Dumbbell Push-ups,** to 5 **Squat Jumps** in place, to 5 **Dumbbell Push-ups** to 5 **Dumbbell Squat Jumps;** repeat 5 times total.

Core: Medicine Ball Twists to Elbows, 10 reps, **to Standing Waist Roll,** 20 reps; repeat 3 times total

Stretch (see pages 58–59)

Dumbbell Split Squat Jumps Forward: Holding a dumbbell in each hand, perform a split squat (bringing one leg out front in a lunge position and bending that leg to 90 degrees). Jump, switching the other foot forward in midair while moving forward, and perform another split squat.

Frog Jump: With your hands on top of your head, squat down to 90 degrees with your legs and rise, hopping forward, two feet at a time.

Dumbbell Push-ups: With a dumbbell in each hand and your body in a push-up position, perform a push-up.

Squat Jumps: With your hands on top of your head, squat downward until your thighs are almost parallel to the ground and your heels remain on the ground. Explode upward, trying to get maximum height.

Dumbbell Squat Jumps: With each hand holding a dumbbell at your side, squat downward until your thighs are almost parallel to the ground and your heels remain on the ground. Explode upward, trying to get maximum height.

Medicine Ball Twists to Elbows to Standing Waist Roll: Lie flat on your back with the medicine ball on your chest, come up 45 degrees, and twist from one side to touch your elbow on the floor, then twist to the other side and do an elbow touch on the floor; do 2 times. Then do a standing waist roll (place hands on hips and roll upper body in hula hoop–like circle).

CLIMBER ▲▲ Weeks 9 and 10 · Monday/Wednesday/Friday

In the drills that follow, you will perform a set of the first exercise (which is sometimes two exercises combined) and immediately follow with a set of the second exercise. Take a few breaths, then repeat each drill twice more. After the 3 sets of each drill, rest for at least 2 minutes before moving to the next one. Your body is being introduced to longer exercise times to prepare and challenge you for future level advancements and longer workouts within the program. Do your best to complete the entire session each day. Your IE session will be a longer one, but try to complete the 2 sets.

1A. **Rocking the Boat,** 20 reps or 1 minute

1B. **Triceps Push-up on Step,** 2 reps, **to Jump over Length of Step,** 10 reps

2A. **3-Point Decline Strap Push-up,** 15–20 reps

2B. **Spider Sprawl to Full Jumping Jack,** 10–12 reps

3A. **Stride to Step Jump,** 8 reps, **to Static Step Jump,** 8 reps

3B. **Strap Core Roll-out,** 15 reps

4A. **Pop-up to Jump with Medicine Ball Overhead,** 12 reps

4B. **Single Leg Squat Upright Cable Row,** 12 reps each arm/side

IE Drill: Complete each drill and then move to the next without rest. Repeat all IEs one more time (H.E.S. 3–4).

1. **Riverdance Training,** 25 yards up and back, 1 time each drill
2. **Animal Sprint Drills,** 25 yards, 5 times up and back for each
3. **Dumbbell Lunge to 2 Frog Jumps Forward,** 25 yards up and back 2 times

Half-Moon Pose; hold for 10 seconds, repeat 3 times total

Lion Pose, hold for 30 seconds

Stretch (see pages 58–59)

Rocking the Boat: Turn the Bosu upside-down and grip opposite sides in push-up position. Lean in one direction and execute a push-up. Switch direction of the lean on each rep.

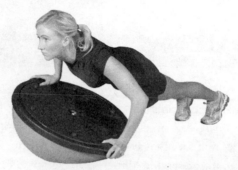

Triceps Push-up on Step to Jump over Length of Step: At the end of a step, do triceps push-ups so the top of your hands almost meets with your solar plexus. Next, squat jump over the entire length of the step. Turn around and repeat the sequence.

3-Point Decline Strap Push-Up: Place one foot in a strap and put your hands in push-up position on the floor, and do a push-up.

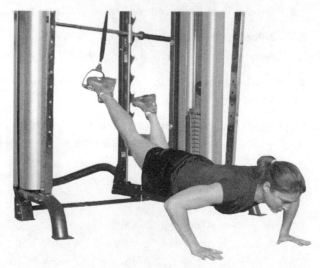

Spider Sprawl to Full Jumping Jack: In push-up position and on your fingertips, pop your feet to under your chest and back down, and then pop them outside line of hands and jump up to a full jumping jack.

Stride to Step Jump to Static Step Jump: Using a step with at least 8 risers, step forward and jump upward onto the step, then jump down. Next, jump from a fixed stance onto the step—taking no forward steps before jumping—then jump down. Raise the step level for each set.

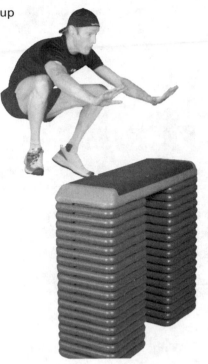

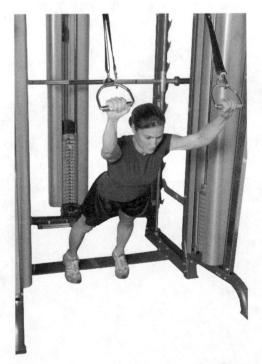

Strap Core Roll-out: In standing position, place your hands in straps and keep them down toward your groin area. Lean forward and let your hands slowly move away from your body until they are almost fully extended and your body resembles a flat V.

Pop-up to Jump with Medicine Ball Overhead: Get into push-up position with hands on top of medicine ball. Pop up quickly, jumping feet to under chest and bringing medicine ball from ground, then jump while bringing medicine ball overhead.

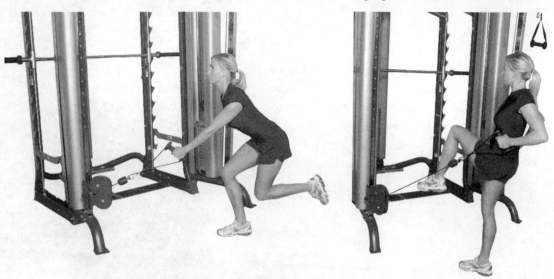

Single Leg Squat Upright Cable Row: Squat on one leg while doing an opposite arm row and bringing your opposite knee up at the same time. Switch sides after the set.

Riverdance Training: Prepare for 5 drills. 1) Run while touching your inside left ankle, and then your right; 2) run while touching outside left and then right; 3) run while touching inside and then outside of your left ankle, and then right ankle; 4) run while kicking, then touching inside your left ankle, outside left ankle, inside right ankle, and then outside right ankle; 5) run while touching inside your left ankle and then your right ankle, to 3 frog jumps with your palms touching floor.

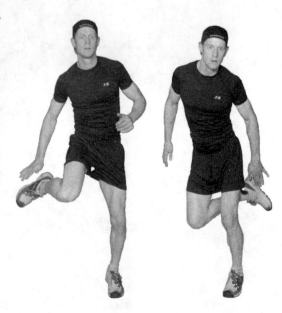

Animal Sprint Drills: Do each of these 3 drills (holding the pose for 5 seconds) before sprinting: 1) start with fingertips on toes; 2) start in a 3-point stance (with one hand elevated); 3) start in a 2-point stance (with one hand and one foot elevated)

Dumbbell Lunge to 2 Frog Jumps Forward: Hold dumbbells at shoulder length during a lunge, then for the first frog jump, hold the dumbbells above your head. For the second lunge, place the dumbbells on the ground between your legs after the jump.

Half-Moon Pose: With your hands on your hips, turn your right knee out with your leg straight and bend your torso to the right while your left leg goes in the air to the left. Bring your right hand to the floor (or use a block if you can't reach the floor comfortably). Your left arm should point straight up, and your left leg should be parallel to the ground, with your left foot flexed. Both your left and right arms should be aligned perpendicular to the ground.

Lion Pose: Sit up on your knees with the heels of your feet pressed against your glutes. Place your hands on your knees, straighten your arms, keeping your back erect and your head straight. Leaning forward slightly and stretching your jaws as wide as possible, extend your tongue out and downward while stretching your fingers straight out from your knees.

CLIMBER ▲▲ Weeks 9 and 10 · Tuesday/Thursday

This workout requires access to a treadmill or grass outside (preferably with hilly areas) (H.E.S. range 2–4).

1. 2-pound cable jump roping, 100 times
2. Place dumbbell in front of you, **Frog Jump** over, grab the dumbbells from between your legs, and place them in front; repeat for 25 yards. Then run backward holding the dumbbells to start
3. With dumbbells between legs, **Frog Jump** forward and alternate between bringing the dumbbells overhead to between your legs; repeat for 25 yards, then run backward holding dumbbells to start
4. **Full Jumping Jacks with Dumbbells,** touching at the top and bottom of movement, 20 reps
5. Repeat numbers 1–4, 4 times total

6. 14% incline run on the treadmill for .25 miles

7. Perform **One-Leg Jumps** over cable rope on floor and back, 10 reps each leg, to **Jump Squat** in place with palms touching the floor, 10 reps. (Keep treadmill running while performing the exercise and then jump back on for the next running series)

8. 12% incline run on the treadmill for .25 miles

9. Perform **One-Leg Jumps** over cable rope on floor and back, 10 reps each leg, to **Jump Squat** in place with your palms touching the floor, 10 reps. (Keep treadmill running while performing the exercise and then jump back on for the next running series)

10. 10% incline run on the treadmill for .25 miles

11. Perform **One-Leg Jumps** over cable rope on floor and back, 10 reps each leg, to **Jump Squat** in place with your palms touching the floor, 10 reps. (Keep treadmill running while performing the exercise and then jump back on for the next running series)

12. Treadmill: 8% incline run for .25 miles

13. Perform **One-Leg Jumps** over cable rope on floor and back, 10 reps each leg, to **Jump Squat** in place with palms touching the floor, 10 reps. (Keep treadmill running while performing the exercise and then jump back on for the next running series)

14. Repeat number 6–13 series 1 more time

15. **Half-Moon Pose:** (with both hands on hips, turn right knee out with leg straight and bend torso to right while left leg goes in air to left; bring right hand to floor—or use block, if you can't reach floor comfortably—left arm to point straight up, and left leg parallel to ground, with left foot flexed; left and right arms should be aligned perpendicular to ground); hold for 10 seconds and repeat 3 times total

16. **Lion Pose:** (sit up on knees with heels of feet pressed against glutes; place hands on knees, straighten arms, and keep back erect and head straight; lean forward slightly, stretching the jaws as wide as possible, extend tongue out and downward, and stretch fingers straight out from knees); hold for 30 seconds.

Stretch (see pages 58–59)

Frog Jump: With your hands on top of your head, squat down to 90 degrees with your legs and rise, hopping forward, two feet at a time.

Full Jumping Jacks with Dumbbells: Holding a dumbbell in each hand, perform a full jumping jack, making sure the dumbbells touch overhead as your legs go out, then touch behind your lower back as your legs come back together.

CLIMBER ▲▲ Weeks 9 and 10 · Saturday

Choose a Recovery Workout provided for you in Appendix D, a recovery workout of your own creation, or a sport-specific recovery workout.

SHERPA ▲▲▲ Weeks 9 and 10 · Monday/Wednesday/Friday

In the 3 intense drills that follow, you will perform a set of the first exercise (which is sometimes two exercises combined), immediately followed by a set of the second exercise, and then a third exercise. Take a few deep breaths and then repeat each drill twice more. After the 3 sets of each drill, rest for at least 2 minutes (or the time it takes to organize equipment for the next drill) before moving to the next one.

1A. **Rough Seas Push-up,** 20 reps

1B. **Ring/Strap Pull-up with Medicine Ball Roll-up,** 10 reps

1C. **Spider Criss-Cross and Dumbbell/Kettlebell Swing,** 12 reps

2A. **Decline Push-up in 3-Point Stance with Knee Lift,** 16 reps (8 reps per leg)

2B. **Skater** back in forth in place 5 reps **to One Leg Jump over Step** with at least 3 risers; repeat (5 skaters then left foot jump over, 5 reps skaters then right foot jump over), 10 reps total

2C. **Burpee Moguls,** 4 reps, **to Half-Ring Spin, to 2 Pull-ups** (with knees up); 12 reps

3A. **Walk-out Fingertip Push-up,** 10 reps

3B. **Barbell Squat, to Biceps Curl, to Step Jump, to Reverse Overhead Press,** 12 reps

3C. **Barbell Squat to Half-Moon** (10 reps each half-moon), 20 reps

IE Drill 1: Repeat the series 4 times (H.E.S. 3–4).

1. **Sideways Push-up Jump to Skaters,** 10 yards, to **Skaters** back to start

2. **180-Degree Squat Jump Spin over Step with Risers,** 10 reps

3. **Backward Frog Jump with Dumbbells,** 20 yards up and back, 3 reps
4. **Spread-Eagle Jump over Step,** 1 rep, **to Daffy Jump over Step,** 1 rep; repeat 10 times

Standing Stability Ball Squats, 20 reps

Stretch (pages 58–59)

Rough Seas Push-up: Turn the Bosu upside-down and grip on opposite sides for push-up position. Place toes on top of the stability ball. Do a push-up in this position.

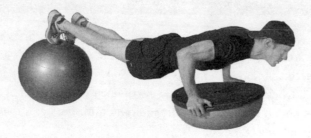

Ring/Strap Pull-up with Medicine Ball Roll-up: With your hands in rings or straps and the medicine ball between your knees, do a pull-up with your palms in, while bringing the medicine ball up toward your chest.

Spider Criss-Cross and Dumbbell/Kettlebell Swing: From a standing position, place your fingertips on the floor with your feet on the outside of your hands and the dumbbell/kettlebell between your hands. Put your feet back, crossing your legs to push-up position, and then immediately pop back, grabbing a heavy dumbbell/kettlebell with both hands, and pulling through overhead.

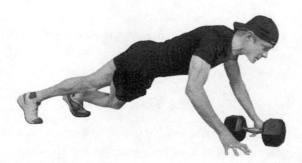

Decline Push-up in 3-Point Stance with Knee Lift: With your hands in push-up position and one foot on a step, do a push-up, then lift the free knee to your opposite shoulder. Switch sides after the set.

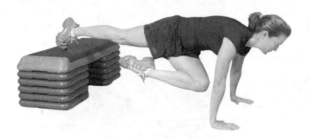

Skater to One-Leg Jump over Step: In place, do 5 Skaters (get into crouch position, like a speed skater; jump to the right, pushing off the floor with your left leg, and land on your right leg. Then immediately push off with your right leg and jump back to land on your left leg; continue until reps are completed), then do one-leg jump over a step with risers, then do 5 more skaters, then jump back over on the same leg. After 5 reps, switch legs.

Burpee Moguls, to Half-Ring Spin, to 2 Pull-ups: Get into push-up position with your feet together and jump your feet together from side to side for 4 reps. Pop up to grab the rings, straps, or a bar with both hands and bring your knees to a 90-degree angle to right side up. Spin your body over and back, and then do 2 pull-ups with your knees remaining up.

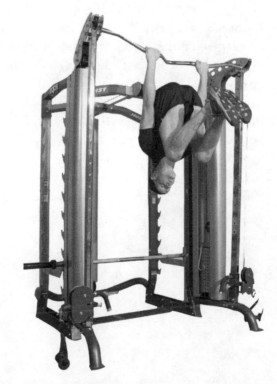

Walk-out Fingertip Push-up: With your feet in rings or straps, walk your hands out until your body forms a push-up position. Raise to your fingertips for 1 fingertip push-up, and then walk back.

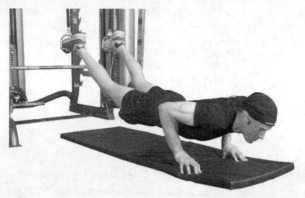

Barbell Squat, to Biceps Curl, to Step Jump, to Reverse Overhead Press: Grab a barbell on the floor with an underhand grip and squat up. Next, curl the barbell and hold it isometrically while jumping onto a step. Once you are there, complete a reverse overhead press. Step down and repeat.

Barbell Squat to Half-Moon: Hold a barbell with weights on the top side with an overhand grip at shoulder level and squat. Next, bend to the side until the bar is almost perpendicular to the ground and the opposite leg is parallel to the ground. Bend back. Switch sides after the set.

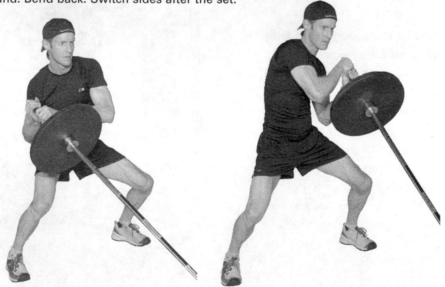

Sideways Push-up Jump to Skaters: Get into push-up position and jump sideways for 10 yards. Pop up and do Skaters (get into crouch position, like a speed skater; jump to the right, pushing off the floor with your left leg and landing on your right leg; then immediately push off right leg and jump back to land on left leg; continue until set is done completely) back to start.

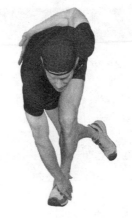

180-Degree Squat Jump Spin over Step with Risers: Stand next to a step with at least 5 risers. Squat and jump over step, turning 180 degrees in midair.

Backward Frog Jump with Dumbbells: Perform frog jumps while moving backward while holding a dumbbell in each hand next to your deltoids, at shoulder level.

Spread-Eagle Jump over Spin to Daffy Jump over Step: Standing in front of a step with at least 5 risers, go down into a squat and touch your palms to the floor, then jump over the step performing a spread eagle (bring legs apart) in midair before landing. Immediately turn around and squat jump again, with your palms touching the floor, and jump back over the step, this time performing a daffy jump (scissoring one leg in front and the other in back) in midair before landing.

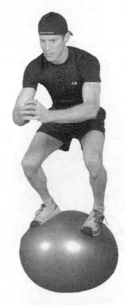

Standing Stability Ball Squats: Using a chair or wall if necessary for balance, place both feet on top of a stability ball and squat.

Use a treadmill or outside grassy trail (preferably with hilly areas) (H.E.S. 2–4).

1. 2% incline warm-up for 5 minutes
2. **Scale the Fence (escape cops left, escape cops right)** using treadmill, 20 reps each, **to Tuck Jump** using treadmill, 20 reps
3. 12% to 15% incline on treadmill for 3 minutes each degree; stay at 15% until you reach 1 mile
4. **Lateral Alien Run,** 20 yards one way; take big breaths and exhale completely until *all* air in your lungs is depleted, then run 20 yards back (stop if you become dizzy or faint)
5. **Treadmill Broad Jump,** 10 reps
6. 12% to 15% incline on treadmill for 3 minutes each degree; stay at 12% until you reach 1 mile
7. **Squat Jump Forward with Barbell, to Overhand Grip Curl-up, to Twist Hits;** repeat 10 times
8. **Squat Jump Forward with Barbell, to Underhand Grip Curl-up, to Twist Hits;** repeat 10 times
9. **Squat Throw Barbell and Catch to Broad Jump Forward;** repeat 10 times
10. 12% to 15% incline on treadmill for 3 minutes each degree; stay at 15% until you reach 1 mile
11. **Lateral Alien Run,** 20 yards one way; take big breaths and exhale completely until *all* air in your lungs is depleted; then run 20 yards back (stop if you become dizzy or faint)
12. **Treadmill Broad Jump,** 10 reps
13. 12% to 15% incline on treadmill for 3 minutes each degree; stay at 12% until you reach 1 mile
14. **Squat Jump Forward with Barbell, to Overhand Grip Curl-up, to Twist Hits,** repeat 10 times
15. **Squat Jump Forward with Barbell, to Underhand Grip Curl-up, to Twist Hits;** repeat 10 times
16. **Squat Throw Barbell and Catch to Broad Jump Forward;** repeat 10 times
17. **Scale the Fence (escape cops left, escape cops right)** using treadmill, 20 reps each, **to Tuck Jumps** using treadmill, 20 reps

18. **Plough Pose**; hold 10 seconds, 3 times total

19. **Cobra Pose**; hold 10 seconds, 3 times total

Stretch (see pages 58–59)

Scale the Fence (escape cops left, escape cops right) to Tuck Jump:
Using a treadmill or chain fence, grab the side rail of the treadmill or the top of the fence. Jump up, bringing your legs parallel to the side rail, and go 20 times to the right and 20 times to the left. Next, jump up, bringing your knees toward your chin, for 20 reps.

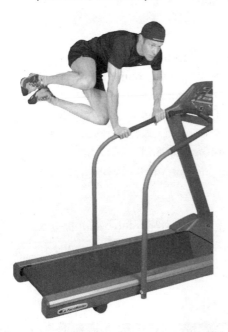
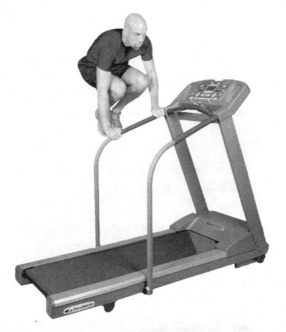

Lateral Alien Run: Go laterally, like a bear, on all fours and with hips staying low.

Treadmill Broad Jump: Facing the treadmill, broad jump over it.

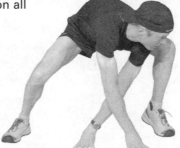

Squat Jump Forward with Barbell, to Overhand Grip Curl-up, to Twist
Hits: Hold a barbell at shoulder level with an overhand grip. Squat jump forward, do a full biceps curl, then twist the barbell to the left and right.

Squat Jump Forward with Barbell, to Underhand Grip Curl-up, to Twist
Hits: Hold a barbell at shoulder level with an underhand grip. Squat jump forward, do a full biceps curl, then twist the barbell to the left and right.

Squat Throw Barbell and Catch to Broad Jump Forward: With a barbell at shoulder level and holding it with an overhand grip, squat down and throw the barbell straight up (make sure your feet come off the ground). Catch, and broad jump forward.

Plough Pose: Lie flat on your back with your legs together and hands palms down by your sides. Raise your legs up and your hips up off ground. Support your back with your hands, keeping your elbows as close to each other as possible. Then, without bending your knees, bring your legs down behind your head. If your feet comfortably reach the floor, walk them as far behind your head as you can and, with toes curled under, push your torso up and heels back. Stretch your arms out behind your back with hands flat on the floor. Breathe slowly and deeply.

Cobra Pose: Lie prone with feet together and toes pointing behind you. Place hands flat on floor and beside rib cage. Gently push off hands, lifting head and chest off ground and tilting head back. Feel chest moving forward as well as upward.

SHERPA ▲▲▲ **Weeks 9 and 10 • Saturday/Sunday**

Choose a Recovery Workout provided for you in Appendix D, a long hike or trail run, a recovery workout of your own creation, or a sport-specific recovery workout for each day.

Chapter 8

REACHING YOUR EVEREST SUMMIT

Weeks 11 and 12

I'D ALREADY SPENT MORE THAN TWENTY-four hours in the "death zone" of Everest, and I knew my body couldn't last much longer. My second and final shot at the summit was that night, when the conditions would determine whether or not I had any prayer of reaching it. After some blustery weather during the afternoon, the sky became clear and the wind died down. It was bitterly cold, at minus 40 degrees, and a steady breeze kept my face frozen solid, even through my space-age head covering—but I felt blessed, because I was being given another chance to go to the roof of the world.

With the half-moon leading me, I struggled at the very beginning of my climb. Trying to find a rhythm, I had to get my body and mind prepared for the daunting overnight task. Frankly, I knew my mind had to take over, because if the decision were up to my body, I'd already be well on my way back to life at lower altitude. Fortunately, while my body was broken, my mind and spirit were willing—greatly aided by the awe-inspiring views over the Himalayas that the moon made possible. The art of high climbing is in systematically moving upward, with very little variation in overall speed. Slowly I found my rhythm and focused on my breathing.

After a couple of hours had passed, however, my muscles began to ache with every step, and my lungs began screeching for more air in order to keep moving. I was nearing the upper troposphere, which is the lowermost portion covering over the earth's atmosphere, and where the most extreme weather phenomena are seen. At 29,000 feet, if an airplane dropped you off without acclimatizing properly, you'd have about 30 seconds before blacking out from the lack of oxygen. Yep, the climb was about to get even tougher.

At that point, the jet stream clouds moved in on me, taking away the moon and the valleys below that had motivated me throughout this final climb upward. Now I was lost in a sea of white. All I could focus on was how worn down my body really was, to the point that falling off the ridge didn't seem like such a bad alternative—anything to end the pain that was beginning to consume me. My body just wanted to rest, nothing else. When I did stop for a few moments, the pain drifted away, but I knew that stopping meant an almost certain death. My engine of survival, my heart, required every bit of blood and oxygen to keep it beating. Therefore, to keep on, my body had no choice—for it had already gone through all the food in my stomach, the glycogen in my muscles, and my fat reserves—but to metabolize my muscle fibers. They were the last energy source in my body, and they were keeping me alive.

Despite all that, I had yet to climb the Hillary Step, a fifty-foot spur of rock, snow, and ice that looms at 28,750 feet. The most well-known physical feature on Everest, the Step is the final significant hurdle on the mountain before it mercifully gives way to angled slopes until the summit. Like all other climbers in modern times, I had access to a fixed rope, but when Hillary and Norgay originally climbed it in 1953, all they had was ancient ice-climbing equipment. Thus they rightfully deserve their homage!

The lack of oxygen and food was exacting a heavy toll, and my lungs had practically given up. Fewer than 100 people have made it to Everest's peak without oxygen, and my goal was to join that elite group. Going to the summit without oxygen wasn't worth dying for, though, so I was taking between 1 and 1.5 liters per minute, which, I found out later, was well below the 3.5 liters per minute of oxygen that is recommended for the death zone (the health editor from *USA Today* told me that taking in so little was worse than not having any supplementary oxygen at all). It was a decision I could live with, though.

I needed every last ounce of strength to pull myself up the Step. The air smelled of the frozen corpses of dead climbers, and it constantly made me want to throw up. I tried to choke my nausea down because I needed to keep all the digestive fluids inside my depleted stomach. I'd had only two liters of water in the previous forty-eight hours, so my body was desperately dehydrated, but my water bottles had frozen, and the process of gathering snow and boiling it would have taken up valuable time.

The wind was only getting harsher, and if I didn't keep up my pace the summit would be lost. I had already seen many guides and their clients turn around, deciding the ascent just wasn't feasible. I was now practically alone, somehow confident I could find the energy and strength to continue. I got my legs underneath me, grabbed my ice ax, and methodically began moving into the pasty clouds ahead with one thought—the summit was up there, somewhere. Reaching Everest's apex flooded every pore that previously had been screaming for me to stop. Finally, after a seemingly endless final push, I arrived at the summit.

The winds were gusting insanely hard. I couldn't stand up for fear of being blown off the mountain, and I had to crouch down on my knees. I couldn't see very far through the clouds. But you know what? I was on the top of the world! My Inner Everest dream had become a reality.

I stood at the summit for three minutes, allowing myself to revel in the achievement. I wanted to stay longer, but there were no picturesque views to be found, the wind was blowing fifty miles an hour, it was 9:30 in the morning, and my job was far from over. Getting down the mountain, in fact, was when many climbers had perished before me, simply too exhausted or too sick from altitude to continue. It turned out that as incredible and life affirming as those few minutes on the summit of Everest were, the descent from the summit to Camp 4 was truly life changing.

Drained of energy, my body experienced the most dangerous sensation—I began to relax. After just having achieved the greatest goal in my life, I realized how much the summit had kept me trudging upward despite having next to nothing in my tank. Now, coming down, I was rapidly losing focus and allowing my weary body to take over my mind. Every five minutes or so, I sat down in the snow to rest and breathe.

And then I got this bizarre peaceful feeling that I might actually die—all I wanted to do was to curl up in the snow and sleep. A crazy thought, perhaps sent by the ghosts of climbers past, came to me, "What a way to go out." But as soon as that occurred to me, I realized that I had far too much to live for and look forward to. Using the Hypermind techniques, I mustered the mental strength to concentrate on what mattered most in my life, where I wanted to be in the future, and how I wanted to get there. I wanted to see my wife desperately, immerse myself in a close-knit community, and start to really live my everyday life to the very fullest. I was just at the beginning of life, not the end! I still had this job I wanted to quit, I still hadn't made all the great changes that were in my mind, and I had so many Inner Everest goals yet to strive for. This wasn't a descent to Camp 4; this was a climb back to life.

While I was destroyed physically, descending Everest without oxygen again connected me with my inner spirit. But just as I thought the weather was going to stabilize, the mountain was hit by a whiteout snowstorm. Rather than panic, I was struck by a very sober thought: that this descent, even after the torturous ascent, was *the* supreme challenge for the human body—and it gave some kind of odd comfort. Without much oxygen left in my lungs, without any sleep or food in three days, with scarcely any water, I had gone well past my limits and was tempting the reaper. But I was no longer afraid.

Because of the inclement weather, other climbers were now hung up at the Step, and I was forced to wait for thirty agonizing minutes. I tried to keep my body moving, but by the time the half-hour elapsed, the interminable snow and wind had entombed my toes in a frozen shell. I knew the results would not be favorable, and the feeling in my fingertips was similarly gone. Yet I retained a sense of confidence—having come this far, and having built this relationship with the mother goddess of the Himalayas—that I was going to make it down alive.

My toes had begun to defrost, bringing with it unimaginable pain. I left my boots on that night because I knew if I took them off, my feet would swell to the size of balloons, and I would be unable to descend to Base Camp on my own steam. I struggled all the way into Base Camp not comprehending the dream goal I had just achieved, and finally got to hug my wife. She claimed she'd never had any doubts, but she kept hugging the skeleton that was me, since I'd lost twenty-five pounds since I'd last been with her, seven days earlier.

Soon I was back at the start of it all, in Kathmandu. Later that night, I felt high on life after having made it to my goal. It had finally begun to sink in. I had reached my Everest, and now I was committed to the idea of helping others reach theirs.

The Game Has Just Begun

You're in the last two weeks of the program, striving toward the finish line. And just like reaching the summit of Everest, many more challenges await. By the end of the twelfth week, hopefully you either will be priming for or have reached your short-term goal, and feel absolutely exhilarated. This is not some simple twelve-week program to get you "over the hump" or one that helps you to "lose those 10 pounds!"—it's much more than that, and it's tougher than that as well. Finishing twelve weeks of Hyperfitness means that you've shown great resolve, and I want you to continue to show your newfound inner and outer strength for the rest of your life.

Reaching your dream will never be easy, especially the Inner Everest goal, but maintaining the Hyperfitness attitude in your mind and heart every day will not only keep you motivated, but it will allow you to triumph over any obstacle that life puts in your way. Remaining focused on your goals during this final portion of the climb is essential, because the combination of fatigue and the prospect of victory being close at hand can cloud your mind and cause you to make a series of mistakes. If you link that short-term goal to the long-term goals that are down the road, then such a letdown will not occur, because you will know you're on a far more significant journey than merely making it through the twelve-week program. Never forget: It's all connected!

Even when your body tires your Hypermind should be restless. In every action you take, ask yourself if it's helping you work toward your goals. Moreover, is it helping you make a difference for the better? You can be watching a movie, sitting down for a leisurely meal, or going to bed at night and still getting your mind to help you along—emptying it of negative thoughts, preparing for future beneficial actions, and simply re-energizing your body for the next workout and the next task.

To reach the big goals, Hyperfitness is a lifetime commitment. So you must turn this twelve-week program into a lifetime of adventure and self-discovery. In this last but crucial self-evaluation, let's find out how ready you are to do that:

- How much better do you feel now than when you started the program more than ten weeks ago?

SECRET SUMMIT TIP

Hyperfitness and Children

By now you know that Hyperfitness not only applies to kids today but that they, in fact, inspire it! With their love of movement, living in the moment, not judging others, and living with absolute curiosity, we can learn a lot from these wonderful, younger versions of ourselves.

Of course, not all of them are such spry, carefree creatures. Rather, many children today are overweight, unhealthy, undisciplined, and stressed out—in other words, they're becoming exactly like a lot of us adults, because they mimic everything we do, and live in a world that we've designed.

More than 9 million American children, or 16 percent, are either overweight or obese. The rate of childhood obesity more than doubled between 1980 and 2000. Are these kids just lazy and gluttonous? Of course not, they're simply following us: the parents!

If you're a parent, you can make sure your child grows up in a healthy environment. Good foods, lots of activity, playing sports, not watching hours of TV or surfing the Internet, not getting too wrapped up in your work or your child's homework, putting family time first, and so on. Being a great parent does take a lot of energy, as well as knowledge about nutrition and exercise. Use Hyperfitness to first inspire you, and then your family as a whole. Share with them how fun it is to be fit, by eating great foods, going on family hikes, playing sports together, exploring the nearest city by foot, and "cardio commuting"—to the library, school, a friend's house, market, pool—whenever you can.

- Can you see the road to changing your life ahead of you?
- How strong and capable do you feel internally right now?
- How has sticking to the Hyperfitness lifestyle changed your mental state and outlook?
- Does your job allow you to express and reveal who you are?
- Are you a passenger or a driver in life?
- Have you come to realize that being fit and healthy is the most precious gift you can give to yourself?

Create a life that not only helps you and others in the near term, but also down the long road . . . for your children and grandchildren and the world as a whole. Here are quotes from two greats in history—I hope they inspire you to think more clearly about your life and the impact it can have.

Avoiding danger is no safer in the long run than outright exposure. Life is either a daring adventure, or nothing.

——HELEN KELLER

The credit belongs to the man who is actually in the arena, whose face is marred by dust and sweat and blood, who knows the great enthusiasms, the great devotions, and spends himself in a worthy cause; who at best, if he wins, knows the thrills of high achievement, and, if he fails, at least fails daring greatly, so that his place shall never be with those cold and timid souls who knew neither victory nor defeat.

——THEODORE ROOSEVELT

These quotes serve to motivate me, especially when I'm discouraged, and they push me back onto the path—the path of Hyperfitness. If I told you eight years ago that I'd be setting world records, standing in front of multinational corporations to give speeches about achieving goals, and also giving back, I'd have said, "No way. I'm the guy who gets embarrassed every time I have to open my mouth

Visualization

Visualization means picturing yourself attaining your goals, no matter what they are. Consistent visualization weaves your dreams firmly into your heart and mind—essential for self-realization.

Before you jump ahead of yourself, take some time, completely on your own—in the middle of the day, before bed at night, or whenever you are unlikely to get interrupted. Get into a relaxed posture, breathe deeply, put on music that makes you feel entirely tranquil, and remain completely in harmony with yourself and your goal, and meditate.

Begin to internalize how you want your actions toward your goal to unfold. The stronger the images, the better chance you have of succeeding. Make your goal visualization extremely detailed and implement as many sensual details as you can—the sight, emotion, smell, and any other sense that can tie you as closely as possible to the vision. Your goal could be an expedition, a race or sports match, a business venture, a potential relationship, or to become adept at a useful hobby or skill, like gardening or carpentry. See yourself doing what it takes, making the right moves, saying the right things, and doing it again and again.

The more positive the visualization, the more likely the outcome will be positive. I imagine myself on the mountain, climbing flawlessly—staying aware of any treacherous conditions, but also taking in all of the natural beauty. I am calm, my body is strong, and I know I will get to where I need to get to that day. Similarly, see your body in the perfect place, doing the perfect things—transferring perfectly from the water to the bike during the triathlon, making the pitch-perfect presentation for a new client, smashing a long drive straight down the center of the fairway, giving a great performance at the act-ing audition, sinking a three-pointer, effortlessly showing the best part of yourself to your date, or simply doing all the Hyperstrength moves with strength and purpose.

The stronger those images are, the better the chance your visualization will come through in your performance. Imagine how your body is feeling, and feel that energy building inside of you. For my speed ascent up Kilimanjaro, I meditated for three to four hours a day with classical music or crashing waves playing on my MP3 player. I saw myself running up the mountain as fast as possible with nothing bothering me; I looked down at my arms and legs going up that mountain with the wind on my face; I envisioned the switchbacks and taking each of them without a problem. By the time I began my ascent, all I had to do was carry out the vision and make sure nothing got in the way.

Once you've got the picture in your head, think of it often—not only when you are relaxing or meditating, but throughout the day as well. This is the process of sending that positive energy out into the universe. I'll start visualizing at least a few months before a major event or expedition, and gradually build until the last few days before showtime, and then it's all I think about.

Finally, believe, with 100 percent of your being, that the goal will be yours.

Along with visualization, practice drills can help your focus and meditation. Lie flat on the ground, and take deep breaths—in through your nose, while your diaphragm expands, and then out through your mouth. Learn to contract each of your muscles individually, and then release completely; start with the crown of the head, then the face, jaw, neck, shoulders, arms, wrists, hands, back, waist, hips, buttocks, thighs, knees, calves, ankles, and feet.

in front of people." I had grown up with few future aspirations or goals that I considered enticing and attainable. I harbored little hope, and lived like a by-stander to my own life. No longer.

You're now on your path, and you know where you want it to take you. You're on your way.

Hyperfare Take-Away Tips

I've covered the major elements of the Hyperfare eating style, but there are some small matters that can add up in the wrong column if you're not aware. There are many popular ingredients, supplements, and habits that I want you to avoid; some are simply a waste of money, but many will do you active harm in both your ability to be healthy and your ability to perform your daily work and workouts.

First, here are **food ingredients to avoid**: trans fats, partially hydrogenated oils, genetically modified corn, excess sugars, high-fructose corn syrup, and ar-tificial flavors. Many of these ingredients are found in processed foods; these products are bad news for your body. They offer many calories, minus the nu-trition that whole food either cooked or eaten raw brings to the table. There-fore, the very simple decision to cook real foods rather than buy processed food will go a long way to making you leaner and healthier.

Second, **don't go crazy with the supplements.** Many people who start working out more frequently and taking their health more seriously consider supplements part of the new game they're playing. Don't be fooled: Many sup-plements are useless, and only exist for their makers to pocket your change. For instance, so many young men are told they need whey protein in order to build muscle, while women are told that they should use a protein drink as a meal re-placement to lose weight. Well, sure, if you were on Mars and didn't have ac-cess to actual food and a kitchen to cook the food in, then, great, go for it. On Earth, though, the only people who should consider taking protein supple-ments are bodybuilders, but even many bodybuilders swear by old-fashioned lean meat and dairy for their protein needs.

The other supplement racket is in so-called thermogenics, which are drinks with an excessive amount of caffeine from various sources. They speed up your heart rate and thus claim to help you lose weight without doing anything and also boost your workout energy.

The only supplement I take is omega-3 fatty acids, which have been proven to block the buildup of inflammatory substances linked to disease and arthritis. Because I don't always eat foods rich in omega-3s—like salmon, mackerel, herring, tuna, and flaxseed—I take the capsule form of fish oil every morning. For the most part you can get everything you need from food, so even a multivitamin is unnecessary. If you're eating a variety of vegetables, fruits, complex carbs, good fats, and quality protein, then you are much of the way there; if you strictly avoid all processed foods (if it comes in a box, you should find out if it is processed), then you're covered. If you're not eating Hyperfare regularly, or are unable to for a period of time (like on a boat trip or on Everest), then I recommend taking a multivitamin.

Most of us really don't get anywhere near a wide enough range of vegetables, sticking mostly to three or four out-of-season vegetables and fruit—such as broccoli, tomatoes, apples, and bananas—meaning they were flown in by jet or brought over on large ships. You might not realize this, but most of the stuff you see in the aisles of your local supermarket falls into this category. Even when we are growing great produce from our gardens in August, the local grocery store usually isn't selling locally grown tomatoes, squash, or onions. When you look closely, you'll notice that it's either from California (even if you live on the East Coast or in the Midwest), Chile, Ecuador, and so on. When food comes from that far away, it doesn't taste as good and it has fewer nutrients. Period. That's why I advocate shopping at farmers' markets where only local growers and producers sell their produce. There are farmers' markets in most cities in the United States these days, and in some of the larger suburban regions as well. I buy and then freeze many vegetables and fruits when they are in season, so when they're out of season our family can still enjoy produce that is still full of nutrition and tastes fresh.

The main caveat is let the buyer beware. Do not simply believe what manufacturers say; their goal is to convince you to buy their product, and to keep using it.

Third, **adjust your eating style.** Sometimes we tend to shovel our food, so before we know it we've eaten more than we need. Instead, savor your food, put down your utensils after each bite, and chew slowly, tasting the flavors. Even if you've worked out like a demon and have raging hunger, take the time to really enjoy your food. It will go so much further, and when you finish you'll find that you're really sated—this might even be the first time you've had this sensation at the end of a meal. Ever notice how "being satisfied" is always paired in TV commercials with a large drink/steak/cookie or some other treat? Advertisers have spent millions persuading us that when something is really big, it tastes better . . . even though the tastiest apple might be the dwarf apple that grows in your aunt's yard, not the waxy monster at the supermarket.

Last, learn how to deal with **"falling off the wagon" episodes,** like food bingeing, drinking too much, and overeating at restaurants. We've all been there, myself included, and it's important not to punish ourselves too severely for one day's mistakes. Having a greasy hamburger, an extra glass of wine, or a big slice of cake once in a while won't kill you, and your physical gains will not diminish because of it. In fact, people who maintain their weight successfully over the long haul are the ones who make constant adjustments for what they ate the day before or at their last meal, almost without having to think about it.

Often stress, depression, or even elation can cause you to binge—as in, "Hey, I need/deserve that huge bowl of ice cream!" With your Hypermind, I hope you'll remember that you may indeed "need" some calories, but there are other important rewards besides food.

Because your Hyperfare plan allows you to eat many great foods and doesn't exclude any type of food (like bread, pasta, or dessert), you will be far less prone to such episodes—and because the Hyperstrength workouts will help you burn more calories than perhaps ever before, you will actually *need* to eat like an athlete and consume a healthy amount of calories.

Hyperstrength, Phase Six:
Weeks 11 and 12

As you enter the eleventh week of Hyperstrength training, you will continue to focus on tandem endurance training and use new phase exercises. All levels will decrease their workout time for the twelfth week—up to 50 percent in time and intensity—to let their bodies rest and recover in preparation for tackling their short-term goals if scheduled immediately after the twelfth week. If not, then forgo the reduction in workout time, and perhaps choose an additional recovery workout in place of a Hyperstrength workout or an extra active day off.

Meredith H., Thirty-one, Sr. Case Management Support Specialist

HF TESTIMONIAL

"I remember the workouts before [the Hyperfitness program], and there is no way I could go back . . .

"In addition to getting a phenomenal physical workout, I also got myself into the right mindset to be able to handle the day's events. I have personally experienced how most things in life are all mental, and your success has to do with what you mentally tell yourself you are or are not able to accomplish.

"Through Sean's Hyperfitness program, at the end of a workout, I reflect back on what I have accomplished and realize that if you set a goal, and set your mind to it, then you can accomplish it. I hear Sean's motivational comments and sayings throughout the day, and any time I have a moment of weakness, feel like taking a shortcut, or doing a substandard job like other coworkers, I realize that if I chose that route I would be no better than the others and would only be cheating myself. At the end of a Hyperfitness day, I have accomplished things that the majority would think were unfathomable.

"I appreciate Sean's program because the work-

outs are always unique and anything but monotonous and routine. The drills from day to day, week to week, month to month, are always different and there is never time to get bored or stagnant within your workout. Every day, more and more, I realize that not only do I enjoy the natural high I get from exercising where I can feel each and every endorphin firing, but I also appreciate the mental workout I receive, which allows me to be in the right frame of mind to have a productive day and to always perform to the best of my ability, especially with the high-stress job I perform.

"I have continued to train in Sean's Hyperfitness program even while pregnant with twins. I now have to go slower due to being pregnant and all the demands pregnancy puts on one's body, which also means modified exercises given by Sean, but all the while the workout still remains challenging and effective. I have no doubt that all the mental training I have learned from Sean's Hyperfitness program inside of and outside of the gym will help me get through labor and delivery."

Mark O., Forty-three, CEO

"**O**ne of the best decisions I have ever made, which has had a major impact on all aspects of my life, was to try one of Sean Burch's Hyperfitness program classes. Little did I know that after sticking it out for several months, it would get me into superior shape, improve my productivity at work and my personal relationships with family and friends, and prove to me that I am capable of setting any goal and meeting it or, more important, exceeding it. I am still Hyperfitness Living seven years and counting."

All levels will perform muscle-building exercises stressing body-weight, free-weight dumbbell, and/or cable exercises, with an additional focus on multiplane functional exercises specific to your particular short-term goal. A Trekker working toward a long weekend kayak or canoe vacation in Maine, for example, can do canoe rows with dumbbells and side twist lunges. A Climber about to embark on a rock-climbing trip in the Catskills might be doing speed skater and rock climber drills, with an optional weight vest. A Sherpa planning a first descent heli-skiing adventure in Alaska might be doing ski mogul masters, including three-point stance knuckle push-ups and jump squats onto steps with risers. This final Hyperstrength phase should be individualized on top of the program I've provided for you, giving you the specific tools needed to conquer your short-term goals.

At the very end of twelve weeks, Trekkers and Climbers can use the self-evaluation portion of Chapter Three to determine whether to progress to the next level or stick with their current programs. I encourage Sherpas to integrate Trekker and Climber exercises into their programs as well to help keep their body off-guard. No matter what your current level, I strongly encourage you to continue your Hyperstrength training, whether that means graduating to the next level or building more slowly.

Overall, keep using Hypermind techniques, Hyperfare nutritional guidelines, and Hyperstrength exercises to keep your mind and body stimulated and challenged after the twelve-week program is finished. No matter what your level, you can move one step closer to achieving your dream goals by going beyond a twelve-week cycle: commit yourself to a life of Hyperfitness.

TREKKER ▲ **Weeks Eleven and Twelve** • **Monday/Wednesday/Friday**

Go straight through the 6 drills below, 3 times, with little to no rest between each complete round of exercises. Your body is being introduced to longer exercise times to prepare and challenge you for future level advancements and longer workouts within the program. Do your best to complete the entire session each day.

1. **3-Point Push-up on Knuckles,** 15 reps
2. **Squat Dumbbell Between Legs to Overhead Press,** for 1 minute 15 seconds
3. **Squat to Jump Medicine Ball Slam,** 20 reps
4. **Canoe Dumbbell Row with Squat,** 10 reps each side (20 reps total)
5. **Squat Dumbbell to Overhead Triceps Extension,** 12 reps
6. **One-Leg Step to Side-to-Side with Medicine Ball Touching Floor to Overhead,** 8 reps on each side (16 reps total)

IE Drill 1: Repeat the drill 3 times total (H.E.S. 2–4).

1. Dumbbells held at shoulder height, **Squat Kick** left/right, 5 reps each leg, place dumbbells down and sprint back and forth touching lines established 20 yards apart, 5 times

IE Drill 2: Repeat the drill 3 times total (H.E.S. 2–4).

1. Run to touching lines 20 yards apart back and forth 2 times, to **Rebounds** (repetitive jumps, as if grabbing rebound, keeping arms overhead), 10 times, to **Bullet Feet** (fast stepping in place), 20 times

IE Drill 3: Repeat the drill 7 times total (H.E.S. 2–4).

1. **Obstacle Course:** Carry medicine ball zigzag-fashion around 4 established obstacles to Jump Squat over step/box, run to endline, **Side-to-Side Squat** while doing big circles with medicine ball back to start of course.

Warrior Pose, 3 times, slow and controlled

Stretch (see pages 58–59)

3-Point Push-up on Knuckles: Get into push-up position with your hands and only 1 foot on the ground; the other remains elevated. On your knuckles, do as many push-ups as possible until 4-point position is needed.

Squat Dumbbell Between Legs to Overhead Press: Hold 1 dumbbell between your legs and squat down. On the way up, swing the dumbbell to shoulder level and press overhead.

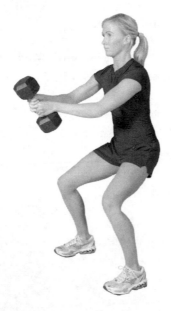

Squat to Jump Medicine Ball Slam: Hold medicine ball at chest height and squat down. Once your thighs are parallel to floor, explode up while slaming ball to the ground.

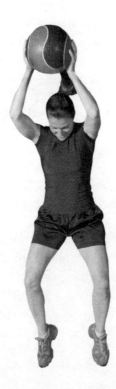

Canoe Dumbbell Row with Squat: Hold a dumbbell in each hand by either side, then squat down and row each dumbbell together once like a rowing canoe. Stand back up and repeat.

Squat Dumbbell to Overhead Triceps Extension: With dumbbells held straight overhead, squat. Bend your elbows and bring the dumbbells toward each other behind your head and press back to straight arms as you come up from the squat.

One-Leg Step to Side-to-Side with Medicine Ball Touching Floor to Overhead: Grab the medicine ball on the floor and bring 1 leg to on top of a step/plyo box. Remain on 1 leg, and push off, jumping over the step while at the same time raising the medicine ball from the floor to overhead. Step down on the other side of the platform, bringing the medicine ball down to the floor. Repeat on the other leg.

Squat Kick: With your feet shoulder-width apart, knees slightly bent, and the dumbbells held in each hand at shoulder height, perform a squat. On the way up, kick your left leg forward and back down. Perform another squat and kick your right leg forward and back down.

Side-to-Side Squat with Medicine Ball Circles: First, point your right shoulder toward the direction you will travel in. Starting with your feet shoulder-width apart and knees slightly bent, descend to a squatting position and swoop the medicine ball to the ground as you begin a shuffle jump to the right. Bring the medicine ball over your head with each shuffle.

Warrior Pose: Take big step forward with your right foot so your right knee is directly over your ankle and your thigh is parallel to the floor. Keep both legs straight and raise your arms forward and overhead. At the same time, bend your right knee to 90 degrees. Next, straighten your right leg and bring your arms back to starting position. Repeat on the left side.

TREKKER ▲ Weeks 11 and 12 • Tuesday/Thursday

Use a stationary bike and a treadmill or outside grass (preferably with some hilly areas) for these drills (H.E.S. 2–3).

1. Warm up for 5 minutes at a slow pace on bike and build up to a moderate pace

2. 1 minute sustained push on bike with medium resistance in seated position to 1 minute of **Pump Clap** (push off handlebars and clap) to 45-second easy spin; or 7% incline run for 2 minutes and then jog recovery at 2% incline for 45 seconds; 3 times total

3. Run up and back 25 yards holding the medicine ball, then do a push-up, then bring medicine ball overhead, 10 times; do series 5 times

4. 1) Shotput medicine ball from one hand back to yourself while moving forward; on the way back switch hands; 2) twist your core with the medicine ball as you run up and back; 3) hold the medicine ball palms up in front of your body, and run up and back; 4) hold the medicine ball like waiter's tray, run up and back; 5) skip while holding the medicine ball at your chest, up and back—25 yards up and back, 3 times each

5. 1 minute sustained push on bike with medium resistance in seated position to 1 minute of **Pump Clap** (push off handlebars and clap) to 45-second easy spin; or 7% incline run for 2 minutes and then jog recovery at 2% incline for 45 seconds; 3 times total

6. Run up and back 25 yards holding the medicine ball, then do a push-up, then bring medicine ball overhead, 10 times; do series 5 times

7. **Squat Medicine Ball Throws** with both hands, straight up from your chest as high as you can throw to one bounce, and repeat; 15 times

8. 1 minute sustained push on bike with medium resistance in seated position to 1 minute of **Pump Clap** (push off handlebars and clap) to 45-second easy spin; or 7% incline run for 2 minutes and then jog recovery at 2% incline for 45 seconds; 3 times total

9. **Split Squat Jump with Medicine Ball** touching left side and right side, 20 reps each side

10. **Warrior Pose:** Take big step forward with right foot, so right knee is directly over ankle and thigh is parallel to floor; keep both legs straight and raise arms forward and overhead; at same time, bend right knee to 90 degrees;

next, straighten right leg and bring arms back to starting position; repeat on left side; 3 times, slow and controlled

Stretch (see pages 58–59)

Split Squat Jump with Medicine Ball: Hold a medicine ball to your chest and assume the split squat position (right foot in front and left in back). Squat down and bring the medicine ball from your chest to the floor on your left side. Once the ball touches the floor, jump up and switch legs, bringing the medicine ball from your chest to the floor on your right side.

TREKKER ▲ **Weeks 11 and 12 • Saturday (Optional)**

Scooter Day!

1. One foot on/off runs (one foot on scooter and push off the floor with the other foot), 5 times; Trekker, Climber, Sherpa
2. V-abs hand pushes (get into V-sit position on a scooter and use only hands to push), 3 times; Trekker, Climber, Sherpa
3. Backward runs (sitting backward on the scooter and using feet only), 4 times; Trekker, Climber, Sherpa
4. Frontward runs (sitting forward on the scooter and using feet only), 4 times; Trekker, Climber, Sherpa
5. Walking and Lunges (place both hands on the sides of the scooter and walk, then lunge left and right), 3 times; Trekker, Climber, Sherpa

---

Scooter Saturday: Trekkers, Climbers, Sherpas

- Be a grown-up child with your child all over again!
- Smooth surface: 30 yards up and back = 1 time

- Perform this series as many times as you like
- Time: Don't worry about it!
- Goal: Embrace your youth!

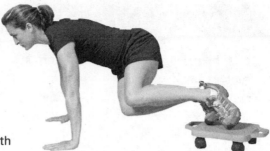

6. Core Diagonals (stationary with hands on floor, feet on scooter diagonally, bring scooter toward your chest and away diagonally), 20 reps; Trekker, Climber, Sherpa

7. Lizard Runs (lie facedown with your navel centered on the scooter; use your hands and feet to move forward), 3 times; Trekker, Climber, Sherpa

8. Push-up (grasp the handles of the scooter in push-up position and do push-ups, max out, 4-point position for Trekkers, 3-point position for Climbers and Sherpas); Trekker, Climber, Sherpa

9. Standing lunge (one foot on the scooter, one foot off, slowly lunge forward extending the leg that is on the scooter into a lunge and back), 10 reps each leg; Trekker, Climber, Sherpa

10. Reverse lunge (foot on the scooter now extends back into a lunge position while the front leg is bent into a squat), 10 reps each leg; Trekker, Climber, Sherpa

11. Arms Push (Use arms only with your knees on the scooter); Trekker, Climber, Sherpa

12. Scooter run 15 yards, stop, Rock Climbers 10 reps, continue 15 yards, 3 reps; Climber, Sherpa

13. Core rolls (grab the sides of the scooter with your hands and roll out the scooter in front of you as far as you can, then pull back in), 10 times; Climber, Sherpa

14. Face-ups (Lying down on your back with your hands on the mat and your knees bent with your feet flat on the scooter, move sideways), 1 time up and back; Sherpa

15. Face-downs (feet are on the scooter while your hands are on the mat; move sideways), 1 time up and back; Sherpa

16. Windshield Wipe (feet are on the scooter; use your hands to move forward while the scooter moves sideways back and forth), 1 time up and back; Sherpa

CLIMBER ▲▲ Weeks 11 and 12 • Monday/Wednesday/Friday

In the 4 drills that follow, you will perform a set of the first exercise (which is sometimes two exercises combined) and immediately follow with a set of the second exercise. Take a few breaths, and then repeat each drill twice more. After the 3 sets of each drill, rest for at least 2 minutes before moving to the next one. Your body is being introduced to longer exercise times to prepare and challenge you for future level advancements and longer workouts within the program. Do your best to complete the entire session each day.

1A. **3-Point Push-up Jump Switch,** 15 reps

1B. **Hands-Down Jump over Step,** 20 reps slow and 20 reps fast

2A. **Cable Swim Backs with Leg Kicks,** 15 reps

2B. **Squat to Alternate Dumbbell Press Overhead,** 10 reps singles, 5 reps doubles

3A. **Donkey Kick to Jump Wide-Grip Pull-up,** 10 reps

3B. **Standing One-Arm Cable Chest Punch,** 10 reps each arm, to One-Arm Push-up on Knees, 5 reps each arm

4A. **3-Point Angled Push-up on Step,** 10 reps each side, **to Jump-over,** 5 reps total

4B. **Side-to-Side Feet with Upside-Down Bosu,** 4 reps, **to Rock Climber,** 4 reps, **to Jump-up and Bosu Throw,** 10 reps

IE Drill: Complete each drill and then move to the next without rest (H.E.S. 2–4).

1. **Squat Jump Forward with Medicine Ball Take-Back**—30 yards up and back, 3 reps

2. 1) Sprint forward to 1-foot leap and land running backward; 2) repeat #1, but keep your hands locked together and behind your body during the run; 3) do a forward to backward leap off one leg, take 4 steps, and then leap from backward to forward running—30 yards up and back, 4 times

3. **Medicine Ball Frog Jump,** 3 reps, to pass medicine ball around core clockwise (up) and counterclockwise (back)—30 yards up and back, 3 times

Hanging Knee-up, max out

Warrior Pose, 4 times, slow and controlled

Stretch (see pages 58–59)

3-Point Push-up Jump Switch: Get into 3-point position (in push-up position with one foot off the floor and other leg elevated) and jump/switch feet after each push-up.

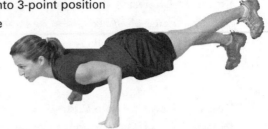

Hands-Down Jump over Step: With your hands down on the top edge of a step with risers or plyo box and your body over the step, jump over the platform with your feet together. Jump back and forth.

Cable Swim Backs with Leg Kicks: Lie facedown on a step with risers placed in the middle of a cable machine, and place a handle in each hand. Be far enough away from the machine so there is tension on the cable. Do the breast stroke with both arms, bringing them wide and behind your body. Meanwhile, perform tiny kicks with your legs behind your body.

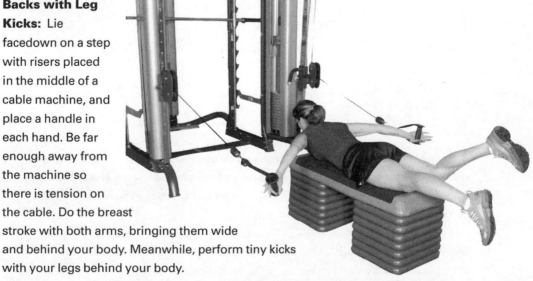

Squat to Alternate Dumbbell Press Overhead: With dumbbells at shoulder level, squat and alternately press one arm at a time (squat each time you press) for 10 reps each. Then squat dumbbell press both arms at the same time for 5 reps.

Donkey Kick to Jump Wide-Grip Pull-up: In push-up position, kick both legs back, and then bring your feet together in front of your chest. Next, jump to grab the pull-up bar with a wide grip and do a pull-up.

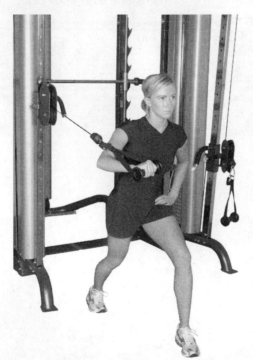

Standing One-Arm Cable Chest Punch: Stand in lunge position and hold a cable handle with one hand. Punch from chest level 10 times, then go down to a one-arm push-up on your knees with the same arm. Switch to the opposite side.

3-Point Angled Push-up on Step to Jump-over: In push-up position with one hand on a step with risers/plyo box and the same side leg elevated, do 10 push-ups. Next, bring your feet together and jump over to the other side and repeat with the opposite arm and leg.

Side-to-Side Feet with Upside-Down Bosu, to Mountain Climber, to Jump-up and Bosu Throw: Turn the Bosu upside-down and get into push-up position with your hands holding opposite sides. Move your feet side to side, 4 times, and then do Mountain Climbers (get into push-up position; keep upper body fixed, then bring right knee to chest and straight again; left knee to chest and straight again; do in staccato, bouncy rhythm), 4 times, and, finally, jump up and bring the Bosu overhead, throw it and catch.

Squat Jump Forward with Medicine Ball Take-Back: Starting with the medicine ball touching the floor, squat jump, bringing the medicine ball up to your chest and out in front, releasing and catching the medicine ball at chest level.

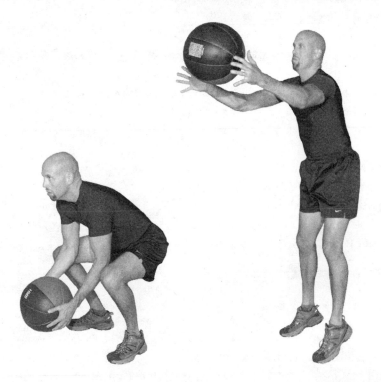

Medicine Ball Frog Jump: Holding a medicine ball to your chest, squat down to a 90-degree angle with your legs and rise, hopping forward, two feet at a time.

Hanging Knee-up: Using a pull-up bar or rings, hang with your arms bent at 90 degrees. Bring your knees to your elbows.

Warrior Pose: Take big step forward with right foot, so right knee is directly over ankle and thigh is parallel to floor; keeping both legs straight, raise arms forward and overhead; at same time, bend right knee to 90 degrees; next, straighten right leg and bring arms back to starting position; repeat on left side.

CLIMBER ▲▲ Weeks 11 and 12 • Tuesday/Thursday

This workout requires access to a stationary bike, treadmill, and/or grass outside. "The Songs Program": perform one drill per song of your choice (H.E.S. 2–3).

1. **Side-to-Side Touching Cones,** 10 yards apart, 20 reps, **to Knee Highs,** 60 reps, repeat for an entire song
2. **Upside-Down Bosu Push-up, to Downward Jumping Jack, to Bosu Jump Overhead Throw and Catch**
3. Jump Rope with 2-pound cable
4. **Knee High Underneath Claps,** 50 reps, **to Full Jumping Jack;** 30 reps, repeat for an entire song
5. **Squat Jump with Medicine Ball,** forward and back 20 yards
6. **Box Jumps** with as many risers as possible
7. **Side-to-Side Medicine Ball Squat**
8. **Daffy Frog Jump to Vertical Jump**
9. Stationary bike spin at light to moderate resistance
10. **Treadmill Incline Push-up to Jump-over**
11. **The Straw** while walking on treadmill at 7% incline or cycling at consistent cadence with low resistance
12. **Warrior Pose,** 4x slow and controlled

Stretch (see pages 58–59)

Side-to-Side Touching Cones to Knee Highs: Stand between 2 cones placed 10 yards apart from each other. As quickly as you can, shuffle back and forth (not letting your feet cross over each other) between the 2 cones, touching the top of each cone with your hand for the allotted number of reps. Next, jog in place, bringing your knees as high as possible.

Upside-Down Bosu Push-up, to Downward Jumping Jack, to Bosu Jump Overhead Throw and Catch: Turn the Bosu upside down and get into push-up position, gripping the sides of Bosu at 3 and 9 o'clock. Perform a push-up. Next, with your hands still on the sides of the Bosu, spread your legs apart fast, and then pop them back together again. Immediately bring your feet together in front of your chest, stand, throw the Bosu overhead, and catch it.

Knee High Underneath Claps: While jogging in place, bring your knees to your chest, clapping your hands underneath your leg with each upward stride.

Squat Jump with Medicine Ball: Squat down with the medicine ball touching the floor, and then jump up, bringing the medicine ball overhead.

Box Jumps: Standing in front of a step with risers, squat and jump onto the step, then step down.

Side-to-Side Medicine Ball Squat: With your feet apart, put the medicine ball between your legs. When your feet are together, move the medicine ball overhead.

Daffy Frog Jump to Vertical Jump: From a standing position, squat and have your palms touch the floor. Then jump straight up performing a daffy jump (scissoring one leg in front and the other in back) in midair before landing. Immediately squat and have your palms touch the floor, then jump straight up as high as possible, bringing your arms overhead.

Treadmill Incline Push-up to Jump-over: Get into a push-up position, with your hands on the side of the treadmill and feet on the floor. Perform a push-up, and then immediately bring your feet together in front of your chest and jump over the side of the treadmill. Turn around and repeat on the other side.

The Straw: Plug your nose and breathe only through a straw. If you become dizzy, immediately remove the straw and breathe normally.

Warrior Pose: Take big step forward with your right foot so that your right knee is directly over your ankle and your thigh is parallel to the floor. Keep both legs straight and raise your arms forward and overhead. At same time, bend your right knee to 90 degrees. Next, straighten your right leg and bring your arms back to starting position. Repeat on the left side.

CLIMBER ▲▲ **Weeks 11 and 12** • **Saturday**

Scooter Day! See page 224.

SHERPA ▲▲▲ Weeks 11 and 12 • Monday/Wednesday/Friday

In the 3 intense drills that follow, you will perform a set of the first exercise (which is sometimes two exercises combined), immediately followed with a set of the second exercise, and then a third exercise. Take a few deep breaths, then repeat each drill twice more. After the 3 sets of each drill, rest for at least 2 minutes (or the time it takes to organize equipment for the next drill) before moving to the next one.

1A. **Upside-Down Bosu Ballistic Spike Push-ups with 2-Point Strap Position,** 15 reps

1B. **Side Jump over Step with Dumbbells,** 16 reps

1C. **Full Rings/Bar Circle to Pull-up,** 8 reps

2A. **Clap Triceps Push-up,** 3 reps, **to 2-Finger Claw Pull-up,** 3 reps; perform 10 reps

2B. **Stand to Squat One-Arm Downward Cable Punch,** 15 reps each arm

2C. **Squat Jump Legs Cross,** 4 reps, **to 180-Degree Dumbbell/Kettlebell Spin,** 10 reps

3A. **Roll-Up Tuck Jump Rear to 2 Pull-ups** (hold last pull-up to 5 seconds); perform 11 reps

3B. **Uneven Push-up, to Pop-up, to 180-Degree Jump over Step,** 20 reps

3C. **Downward Jumping Jack,** 2 reps, **to Jack Rabbit,** 2 reps, **to Toes/Fingers Touch Jump,** 2 reps; perform 12 reps

IE Drill: Repeat the series 4 times (H.E.S. 3–4).

1. **Dig Shovel Jumps,** 30 reps each side
2. **Tuck Jump with Towel Touching Toes,** 15 reps slow, 5 reps fast
3. **Crabwalk** for 20 yards, **to Diagonal Foot Bounds, to Medicine Ball Throw Behind Head** against wall, 5 reps; perform 7 reps

Standing Stability Ball Squats, 20 reps

Warrior Pose, 4 times, slow and controlled

Stretch (see pages 58–59)

Upside-Down Bosu Ballistic Spike Push-ups with 2-Point Strap Position: Turn the Bosu upside-down and get into push-up position by gripping at 3 and 9 o'clock, while putting one foot into a strap. For each push-up, push off the ground as high as possible and then all the way down to your chest. Switch feet in the strap next round.

Side Jump over Step with Dumbbells: While holding dumbbells, side jump over a step with risers.

Full Rings/Bar Circle to Pull-up: Do a full rings/bar circle (hold rings or bar with arms and legs bent at 90 degrees; twist body over your head and then back so 180 degrees is covered), then pull your body up with palms facing each other to a complete pull-up. Feet never touch the floor throughout all reps.

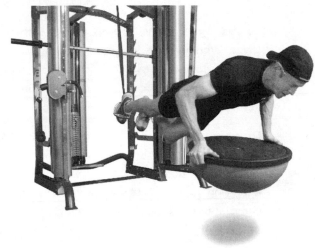

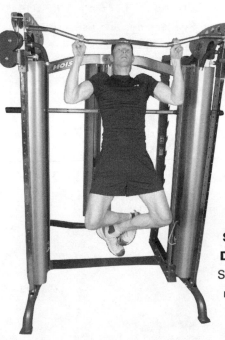

Clap Triceps Push-up to 2-Finger Claw Pull-up: Get into triceps push-up position and explode off the ground to clap hands, 3 reps, then pop your feet under your chest and jump up to grab the pull-up bar. With the first two fingers only, pull up twice.

Stand to Squat One-Arm Downward Cable Punch: Hold the cable, hand at chest level beside your body. Squat down and punch straight down.

Squat Jump Legs Cross to 180-Degree Dumbbell/Kettlebell Spin: Squat jump and then cross/uncross legs in midair, landing in place. Then grab a kettlebell or dumbbell and squat jump, turning 180 degrees in the air.

Roll-up Tuck Jump Rear to 2 Pull-ups: Lie on your back and roll your body up (bring arms from overhead to roll up, one vertebra at a time while legs are bent) and stand. Jump, bringing your heels to your glutes. Next, grab the pull-up bar. Do 2 pull-ups, holding the last pull-up for 5 seconds.

Uneven Push-up, to Pop-up, to 180-Degree Jump over Step: With one arm on a step with risers or a plyo box and the other on floor, and both feet on the floor, do a push-up and then pop your legs under your chest and do a 180-degree jump over the platform. Repeat on the other side.

Downward Jumping Jack, to Jack Rabbit, to Toes/Fingers Touch Jump: Do a downward jumping jack (in push-up position, shoot your legs apart). Pop feet back to push-up position and bring your heels to your glutes. Then bring your feet together in front of your chest, stand and tuck jump, bringing your toes to your fingertips to touch in front of you while in midair.

Dig Shovel Jumps: With a weighted bar, start in a squat position with the bar near your right ankle with a left underhand grip first, then right overhand, gripping the bar behind. Squat jump forward, bringing the bar diagonally across your body and over your left shoulder. Repeat. Switch sides and use a right underhand grip first, then left hand overhand grip behind it.

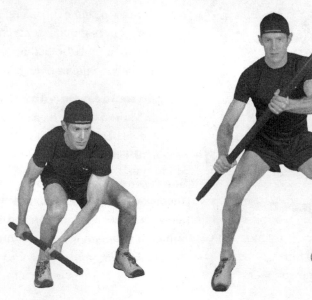

Tuck Jump with Towel Touching Toes: Holding a towel in your hands, tuck jump and bring your toes to the towel in midair.

Crabwalk, to Diagonal Foot Bounds, to Medicine Ball Throw Behind Head: Your body is facing upward with hands and feet on the floor moving forward for 20 yards. Then do one leg diagonal bounds forward from left to right leg forward touching the outside of the lead foot with the opposite hand each time back to start, and then cock the medicine ball behind your head with both hands and fire against a wall (do not release the ball if there is no wall). Catch, and repeat the sequence.

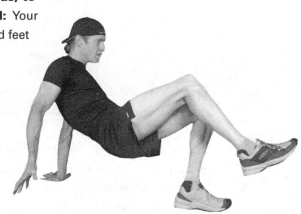

Standing Stability Ball Squats: Stand on a stability ball, squat down until thighs are parallel to ground, then squat back up.

Warrior Pose: Take big step forward with right foot, so right knee is directly over ankle and thigh is parallel to floor; keeping both legs straight, raise arms forward and overhead; at same time, bend right knee to 90 degrees; next, straighten right leg and bring arms back to starting position; repeat on left side.

SHERPA ▲▲▲ Weeks 11 and 12 • Tuesday/Thursday

Use a stationary bike, treadmill, and/or outside grass (preferably with hilly areas). Follow "The Songs Program #2," performing one drill per song (H.E.S. 2–3).

1. Jump over Bosu side to side with medicine ball overhead to touching floor
2. With hands on the top edge of a step with risers or plyo box, and your body over the step, jump over the platform with your feet together, jumping back and forth, 10 times slow, 40 times fast, to Full Jumping Jacks, 20 reps; repeat for one song

3. **Roll-up Tuck Jumps Rear** (sing the song playing out loud for its entirety)
4. **Bouncing One-Leg Straight Kick,** 10 yards, **to Jump-up** to step with risers or plyo box (at least 3 feet high)
5. Jump rope with 4-pound cable, 30 seconds on, 15 seconds off
6. **Box Jumps** over steps with at least 10 risers or plyo box, holding at least 20-pound dumbbells
7. Ski Mogul Master to 2 Full Sit-ups
8. **Heavy Medieval Bastard Slam, to Triceps Push-up, to Downward Jumping Jack, to Jump-up with Heavy Medieval Bastard Overhead;** repeat
9. **Frog Jump with Heavy Medieval Bastard Circle** (sing the song playing out loud for its entirety)
10. Stationary bike spin at light to moderate resistance
11. Repeat drills 1–10 one more time
12. **The Straw** with treadmill incline walk at 12% incline or cycle at low resistance with consistent cadence for 5 minutes
13. **Warrior Pose,** 4 times, slow and controlled

Stretch (see pages 58–59)

Roll-up Tuck Jumps Rear: Lying on your back, roll up as fast as you can to your feet and jump up quickly, bringing your heels to your glutes in midair before landing on your feet.

Bouncing One-Leg Straight Kick to Box Jump: Stand with your hands on top of your head. Bounce forward on one leg while kicking straight out in front of you with the opposite leg up. Next, squat and jump onto a step with risers (or plyo box), then step down on the other side.

Heavy Medieval Bastard (HMB) Slam, to Triceps Push-up, to Downward Jumping Jack, to Jump-up with Heavy Medieval Bastard Overhead: Hold the HMB (medicine ball) at chest height and squat down. Once your thighs are parallel to the floor, jump up, bringing the ball over your head and slamming it to the ground. Next, place both hands on the HMB, get into a push-up position, and perform a triceps push-up. Then, keeping your hands on the HMB, spread your legs apart and pop your legs back together again. Immediately bring your feet together in front of your chest, stand, and jump straight up as high as possible, bringing the HMB overhead before landing.

Frog Jump with Heavy Medieval Bastard Circle: Hold an HMB (medicine ball) to your chest, squat down to 90 degrees with your legs, and rise, hopping forward, two feet at a time, while bringing an HMB around in a circle rotation in front of your body.

The Straw: Plug your nose and breathe only through a straw. If you become dizzy, immediately remove the straw and breathe normally.

Warrior Pose: Take a big step forward with your right foot so that your right knee is directly over your ankle and your thigh is parallel to the floor. Keep both legs straight and raise your arms forward and overhead. At same time, bend your right knee to 90 degrees. Next, straighten your right leg and bring your arms back to starting position. Repeat on the left side.

SHERPA ▲▲▲ **Weeks 11 and 12** • **Saturday/Sunday**

Scooter Day! (See page 224.) Sunday is an active recovery day.

YOUR HYPERFITNESS LIFESTYLE

WITHIN TWO MONTHS OF CLIMBING Mount Everest, I quit my day job, began a new career in motivational speaking and fitness consulting, and carried on with my personal and group training business. I could see the way ahead of me: It no longer meant being a world beater, but rather making the world better. To do this, without even realizing it at the time, I set out on the path of Hyperfitness—discovering the keys to building a life of passion and purpose along the way.

There was, is, and always will be plenty of work to be done to address the issues of poverty, genocide, starvation, the growing disparity between the rich and the poor, environmental degradation, and simply surviving wars, let alone ending them. When considering these abiding problems, it is difficult not to respond with sadness and hopelessness. What can one do?

It's imperative not to simply throw up your hands in despair, though; wrap them (as well as your mind) around positive ideas and vow to change things, even if your success moves at the speed of one person at a time. The more you define the problem, the more you can define the solutions, just like in our self-evaluations.

How come I've brought all this up in a fitness book? I believe it's because all good things in your life and in the lives of others you touch begin with a healthy mind and body. Exercise and the expeditions I went on saved me from leading a life that would have been meaningless. Hyperfitness got me into amazing shape, but much more than that: It connected me to what my life really should be about.

The Hypermind, Hyperfare, and Hyperstrength programs will serve you in the same manner, by giving you far more than the "bathing suit body" or the "leaner, meaner me." Those are very legitimate goals—just as is developing into a great athlete (which will happen with this program, even if you don't want it to!)—but you've learned to set goals in every area of your life.

You've heard my students testify about how Hyperfitness helped them overcome enormous obstacles and achieve remarkable goals. You've read how Hyperfitness transformed me, body and soul, into someone who could run a world record–breaking marathon at the North Pole and break the world record ascent for Mount Kilimanjaro, while still attending to the needs of my growing family. You are no different! You now have the tools to scale the summit of your own Inner Everests.

Reaching Your Peak

How far will you go up the mountain toward your short-term goals and long-term goals? I've told you how to attain your dream goals, so now it's up to you to go out in the real world and do everything in your power to accomplish them. Don't be the person who reads but does not retain, who listens but refuses to act, who sees the goal but fails to follow through.

Are you in the driver's seat yet? A friend of mine in college hated to drive. Every time any of the guys went out, he'd be the first to yell, "Shot-gun!" just so he wouldn't have to drive. Half the time he'd sleep in the car or zone out until we reached our destination, while the rest of us talked or listened to music. A passenger may think they have the better seat because they don't have the responsibility of keeping their eyes on the road, staying focused, alert, and ready; they just sit back and watch the world go by. Be in control of your own destiny.

Imagine yourself in your very advanced years, reminiscing about your life and adventures with your spouse or friends. During those moments, would you have any reservations about your past and wish you had pursued something in particular, gone somewhere special, or persevered through a difficulty that still affects you? Or do you wish you had chosen a more idealistic path? I want you to be able to look back without regrets, having lived without any self-imposed boundaries.

To keep yourself centered and focused on fulfilling your envisioned plans, take the solo self-discovery journey every now and then. Use the time you spend in each Hyperstrength workout to strengthen your mind and cleanse your soul. Take in renewed energy and love for life during every Hyperfare meal. And, no matter what, never stop questioning, learning from, and, ultimately, embracing what each day brings you.

When I first step outside my house in the early morning on the way to teach a Hyperfitness class, I make it a habit to look up at the sky and stars. I imagine what it must be like for those astronauts to orbit the Earth and see the immense beauty of our blue planet staring them in the face. This is a new day. No one owns it yet, and this day could be mine, where I make my dreams come true. I ask myself: Is today the day I improve someone's life forever? Is today the day I make the world a better place to live?

If I had turned around before reaching the summit, like so many of my fellow Everest climbers on that brutal day in May of 2003, no one would have blamed me. I still would have met my quota and lived up to everyone's expectations—but I was capable of more. Deep down, to the very marrow of my bones and to the depth of my soul, I knew that I could achieve the summit of Everest and return safely back to Base Camp. There wasn't an expedition leader showing me the way. It was up to me, and only me, to decide my fate.

Similarly, let your future be decided by you. You're now at a point where your goals make you feel truly alive, so keep gaining on them. Take what God has given you and use every ounce of it.

Live Simple, Live Boldly

Sometimes you will struggle to make it work and feel overwhelmed by family, work, dire current events, debt—the list goes on and on. Stressful and traumatic situations can knock us off our stride, and then we are also assaulted on a daily basis by conventional nuisances such as being told what we need to buy, look like, visit, live, possess, and on and on.

The answer? Simplify your life. When I returned from Everest, I was desperate to quit my job because it didn't provide any meaning to my life. But because my boss had believed in me and let me take time off of work for my expeditions, I couldn't leave her hanging; so I cut down my hours and subsequently lost my benefits. Suddenly my family and I had to do with less, and it was not just enough—it was better. I had worked for years in a soul-destroying job, for what? So I could keep up with the Joneses, or maybe even surpass them? So I could afford expensive restaurants, luxurious automobiles, and high-priced toys? Don't get me wrong; it's wonderful to have wealth and security, but was that all I wanted out of life? I felt like the trapped American who didn't think he had a choice, did not think he could make a difference in the world. I told myself, "That's the way life is." That's bullshit. Life is wonderful if you allow yourself the freedom to live it on your terms—to pursue your dreams with passion and bring good to others at home and throughout the world. Is that a lofty ambition? Sure. But nothing of great meaning begins with anything else.

We all have serious obligations, especially if we're supporting a family, so we can't just chuck the job and start pounding away on our bongos at home. But there is nothing preventing you from creating goals—like getting a promotion, switching careers, learning to speak a foreign language, swimming across the English Channel, or altering your social or political climate—that will make the future a lot more desirable and fulfilling than your current existence. If you feel the pull toward something that you are meant to do, then heed that call and start planning for it now.

As you approach your goals and as your life grows, you inevitably will encounter some challenging transitions. These can be more easily managed if you boil down your life to the basics. For me, it's family and work that I love, exercise and nutrition that I need, and spirituality that keeps it all together. No matter what curveball life throws me, I can deal when I return to these roots of strength.

After I had climbed my first reputable mountain, I became a mountaineer. I believed with all my heart that I would one day climb Everest, because I was now a mountaineer. Ever since I was eight years old I dreamed about writing a book—but I never believed it could happen until after I climbed Everest.

Instead of doubting, and stifling your hopes in yourself, believe the best about yourself. Watch your belief blossom and strengthen with every workout, every healthy meal, and every little goal you achieve—until you're close to reaching the big goals and becoming what you believe.

The old adage that nothing worth doing is easy really is true. But it's also true that if it's worthwhile, then it's worth the sweat and the struggle—and that the rewards are beyond compare. I congratulate you on committing to the Hyperfitness program over the past twelve weeks. Keep on, be brave, change the world.

Skål,
Sean

HYPERFARE MEALS AND RECIPES

Breakfast

Quick Breakfast

KICKSTART METABOLISM • Serves 1

1 to 2 cups GOLEAN Cereal with 8 ounces nonfat organic milk and ½ cup
blueberries or blackberries

Other cereal alternatives: Back to Nature Flax & Fiber Crunch, Nature's Path
Organic Flax Plus

1 slice whole-wheat toast with all-natural peanut butter

THE LEAN ELVIS • Serves 1

2 slices seven-grain bread with all-natural peanut butter and slices of ½ banana

6 ounces organic low-fat fruit yogurt with slices of the other ½ of banana and a
handful of frozen blueberries

NORWEGIAN SPLENDOR • Serves 1

1 organic whole-wheat pita stuffed with low-fat cream cheese spread and 3 ounces Norwegian smoked salmon, 1 tomato slice, 1 red onion slice, and a half dozen capers sprinkled on top, topped with a dash of red pepper flakes and a squeeze of lemon

Cooked Breakfast

THE BRAWN OMELET • Serves 1

Organic olive oil spray
2 teaspoons crushed garlic
¼ cup chopped portobella mushroom
¼ cup chopped spinach leaves
3 chopped plum tomatoes
4 egg whites
6 ounces chopped cooked skinless chicken or turkey (leftovers from another meal)
Pinch of dried oregano
Nonfat sour cream, for serving (optional)
Chipotle salsa, for serving (optional)

◆ Coat a medium nonstick pan with olive oil spray and place over medium heat. Sauté the garlic and vegetables for 5 minutes or until softened. Pour the egg whites into the pan and add the chicken or turkey. Cook the egg whites until cooked through, then add the oregano. Fold over the omelet, take off the heat, and cover for 3 to 5 minutes.

◆ Serve with a dab of sour cream and/or chipotle salsa.

RECOVERY WRAP • Serves 1

Organic olive oil spray
1 small chopped onion
½ cup yellow or red bell peppers
¼ cup sliced portobella mushrooms

1 whole egg plus 2 egg whites, beaten

1 whole-wheat tortilla

¼ cup part-skim mozzarella

3 dashes of Cajun spice

1 tablespoon prepared salsa

◆ Coat a medium nonstick pan with olive oil spray and place over medium heat. Sauté the vegetables for 5 minutes, or until softened, remove from the pan, and set aside. Spray the pan with olive oil spray again, add the egg and whites, and scramble until set. Place the scrambled eggs and vegetables on a whole-wheat tortilla, spinkle with the mozzarella cheese, Cajun spice, and salsa. Roll up the tortilla.

Lunch

Quick Lunch

TURKEY TROTTER • Serves 1

An open-faced sandwich with a slice of toasted organic sprouted grain bread topped with 6 ounces of smoked turkey breast, 1 thick tomato slice, ¼ cup chopped cooked shiitake mushrooms, a small handful of mesclun, and finished with honey-mustard or all-natural vinaigrette

Vegetable salad and/or organic apple on the side

VEGANS RULE • Serves 1

A cracked-wheat hamburger bun spread with a small layer of store-bought or homemade hummus and topped with grilled vegetables (1 thick slice of organic portobella mushroom, 1 slice organic eggplant, and 1 organic zucchini, sliced lengthwise) and sprinkled with your favorite hot sauce of black pepper.

MANDAL HEAVEN • Serves 1

½ organic whole-wheat baguette, cut in half and topped with: 1 sliced cucumber, ½ sliced avocado, 6 peeled shrimp, 1 sliced hard-boiled egg, 1 teaspoon chopped fresh dill, a squeeze of lemon, and a dash of salt and pepper.

Cooked Lunch

AT FIGHT WEIGHT QUESADILLA • Serves 1

½ teaspoon extra-virgin olive oil
1 tablespoon crushed garlic
1 cup cooked black beans
1 whole-wheat tortilla
¼ cup grated part-skim mozzarella
½ cup chopped cooked yellow squash
Dash of hot sauce

◆ Warm the olive oil in a small sauté pan over medium heat. Add the garlic and sauté until softened, about 2 minutes. Add the beans and cook until warmed through. Spread the beans over the tortilla and top with the mozzarella and squash. Fold the tortilla and serve with the hot sauce. Serve with an organic apple on the side.

THE ENERGY MAINTAINER SALAD • Serves 1

1 cup cooked organic quinoa, chilled
8 ounces of wild skinless, boneless pink salmon
1 finely chopped carrot
1 finely chopped scallion
1 sliced cucumber
1 diced tomato
½ cup steamed spinach
¼ cup crumbled feta cheese

¼ avocado, sliced

Small handful of sprouts

Small handful of watercress

1 teaspoon ground turmeric

Pinch of cayenne pepper

Fat-free balsamic vinaigrette

◆ Mix all the ingredients together in a bowl. Drizzle the vinaigrette on top. Have a handful of organic granola for dessert.

HEALTHY DAMN HOT WINGS • Serves 1

4 tablespoons hot sauce, plus more for serving

1 tablespoon honey

2 tablespoons Dijon mustard

8 ounces skinless chicken tenders

◆ Whisk together the hot sauce, honey, and mustard in a small bowl. Place the chicken tenders in a zip-top bag, add half the sauce, seal, and marinate in the refrigerator for 3 hours. Heat a medium nonstick skillet over medium heat. Remove the chicken from the marinade and cook until white inside, turning once and coating the chicken with the remaining sauce during the last 5 minutes. Top with hot sauce to taste and serve with fat-free blue cheese, organic baby peeled carrots, and a glass of organic skim milk.

Quick Sides

POWER LUNCH SIDE • Serves 1

1 baked sweet potato (with skin), topped with ¼ cup shredded part-skim mozzarella, ¼ cup chopped broccoli, and a dollop of all-natural nonfat sour cream

HEALTHY FRIES • Serves 2

◆ Cut 2 sweet potatoes (with skin) into strips and place on a baking sheet sprayed with organic olive oil spray. Sprinkle with Old Bay seasoning and bake at 425°F for 15 to 20 minutes, or until nicely crisp. Serve with organic ketchup.

Dinner

FEEL-GOOD CALAMARI SOUP • Serves 1

2 tablespoons organic extra-virgin olive oil

8 ounces cleaned squid

1 teaspoon garlic powder

½ teaspoon cumin

¼ teaspoon ground nutmeg

Dash of cardamom

Dash of cinnamon

Dash of turmeric

Dash of freshly ground black pepper

Juice of ½ lemon

16 ounces organic vegetable broth

3 of your favorite vegetables, such as organic broccoli, tomatoes, or
    asparagus, sautéed

◆ Heat 1 tablespoon of the olive oil in a medium sauté pan over medium heat. Add the squid and sauté for 4 minutes, or until cooked through. Set aside.

◆ Combine the garlic, cumin, nutmeg, cardamom, cinnamon, turmeric, black pepper, and lemon juice in a bowl. Add the remaining 1 tablespoon olive oil and stir to combine. Add the squid.

◆ Place the vegetable broth in a medium saucepan and heat until hot. Add the squid, and sautéed vegetables (three favorite seasonal vegetables) to the broth and cook for 1 minute, then serve.

BHS CHILI • Serves 2

1 chopped onion

5 finely chopped garlic cloves

14-ounce can organic chopped tomatoes or 5 medium fresh chopped
   organic tomatoes

32 ounces organic chicken broth

2 teaspoons ground cumin

15-ounce can kidney beans, drained

2 tablespoons of hot pepper flakes, or to taste

½ cup chopped jalapeño chiles, or to taste

½ tablespoon ground chipotle chile

Hot sauce, to taste

1 pound ground venison

◆ Sauté onion and garlic in a large pot. Add tomatoes, chicken broth, cumin, beans, hot pepper flakes, jalapeños, and ground chipotle. Bring to a simmer over high heat, then reduce the heat to low and cook for 20–30 minutes.

◆ Meanwhile, cook the venison in a medium saucepan over medium-high heat until it is cooked through and light pink. Add the venison to the chili just before serving.

WILD SALMON VEGETABLE MEDLEY • Serves 2

½ tablespoon honey

Juice of 1 lemon

1 teaspoon light soy sauce

½ tablespoon organic whole-grain mustard

½ tablespoon crushed garlic

One 16-ounce wild Pacific salmon fillet

◆ Preheat the oven to 375° F. Combine the honey, lemon juice, soy sauce, mustard, and garlic in a small bowl.

◆ Brush the salmon with the mixture. Wrap in aluminum foil and bake until light pink, about 20-30 minutes. Serve with your favorite steamed vegetables.

HYPERSTRENGTH PROTEIN SALAD • Serves 2

1 cup of cooked organic quinoa, chilled

Half a head of romaine lettuce

2 sliced organic tomatoes

2 sliced red bell peppers

1 sliced cucumber

1 chopped carrot

½ chopped onion

½ cup cooked organic black beans, drained

2 6-ounce cans Tongol light tuna

2 hearts of palm

2 tablespoons Trader Joe's Sesame Soy Ginger Vinaigrette

Hot red pepper flakes, for serving

◆ Combine all ingredients in a large bowl.

THE LEAN AND DEFINED • Serves 1

◆ Grill your choice of meat (8 ounces of skinless, boneless, organic chicken breast, antelope, or venison) until light pink, seasoning with dashes of salt, pepper, and oregano. Steam 2 cups of your choice organic cauliflower, carrots, yellow squash, peas, and/or broccoli. Serve with 1 steamed artichoke or artichoke hearts marinated in low-fat raspberry vinaigrette.

SATURDAY COPS PIZZA • Serves 2–4

1 pound packaged whole-wheat pizza dough, rolled out into desired shape pizza

1 cup prepared organic tomato sauce

1 orange, green, or red bell pepper, sliced

1 tablespoon dried oregano

1 tablespoon Old Bay seasoning

½ cup steamed spinach

12 ounces ground or diced venison, buffalo, or shrimp

½ cup sliced portobella mushrooms

¾ cup grated part-skim mozzarella or organic low-fat cheddar cheese

◆ Set the oven dial at 425° F, and immediately put the rolled-out dough into the oven for 10 minutes. Once oven is preheated, take out dough and add all the ingredients except the meat. Place back in oven, raise the temperature to 475° F for 10 minutes, then remove and add the meat to the pizza, place back in the oven, turn off the oven, and leave until the meat is cooked through, about 5 minutes.

THE POWER BURGER • Serves 3

1 pound of ground buffalo or venison
1 finely chopped onion
1 teaspoon ground tumeric
1 teaspoon ground cumin
1 teaspoon cayenne pepper
1 teaspoon garlic powder

◆ Mix together the meat with the onion and spices and form 3 patties. Cook for 10 minutes, flipping halfway through.
◆ Top with a thick organic tomato, organic yellow onion slices, and mixed greens. Serve in an organic whole-wheat pita pocket with your favorite condiment (such as chipotle salsa, mango chutney, or wasabi sauce).

THAMES CHICKEN • Serves 2

12 ounces organic skinless chicken breast, cut into strips
Squeeze of lemon and lime
2 finely chopped chiles
1 teaspoon chopped fresh basil
1 teaspoon chopped fresh ginger
1 teaspoon chopped fresh cilantro
8 ounces Pad Thai noodles, uncooked
⅓ pound chopped organic asparagus
½ cup chopped shiitake mushrooms
1 chopped spring onion
⅓ pound organic green beans, trimmed

◆ Marinate the chicken for 30–45 minutes with the lemon juice, lime juice, and spices and then stir fry until completely cooked. Set aside. Boil noodles until soft. Drain and set aside. Sauté the asparagus, mushrooms, spring onion, and green beans until al dente and toss to combine with the chicken and noodles.

POWER DINNER SIDE • Serves 1

◆ Combine ½ cup cooked whole-wheat couscous or 4 ounces cooked organic whole-wheat penne with olive oil; minced garlic, ground pine nuts, fresh basil leaves, and a pinch of black pepper.

Smoothies

ANTIOXIDANT BERRY BLAST • Serves 1

Blend together:
1 cup nonfat organic milk
6 ounces organic low-fat plain yogurt
½ cup strawberries
½ cup blueberries
½ cup blackberries
½ cup raspberries
6 ice cubes, or more as needed

ENERGY KING • Serves 1

Blend together:
1 cup nonfat organic milk
1 tablespoon organic honey
1 cup organic low-fat berry yogurt
1 cup frozen mangoes
1 teaspoon crushed flaxseed
4 ice cubes

PROTEIN PUMP • Serves 1

Blend together:

½ cup organic vanilla soymilk

8 ounces nonfat vanilla yogurt

A few dashes of ground cinnamon

1 tablespoon organic almond butter

¼ cup organic rolled oats

6 ice cubes

Desserts

- 1 banana sliced with a drizzle of organic chocolate syrup
- Frozen berries, sliced banana, mango, or other fruit. My favorite is frozen red grapes
- Hansen's Diet natural root beer with 1 scoop organic nonfat vanilla frozen yogurt
- 6 ounces organic low-fat strawberry yogurt with ½ frozen banana, chopped
- 1 organic piece of seasonal fruit with 1 scoop organic nonfat ice cream

Condiments

NUMERO UNO SALSA

◆ Besides being low in calories, salsa contains ingredients that are full of nurturing compounds such as flavonoids, lycopene, and carotene.

1 tomato, finely chopped

¼ cup diced jalapeño chiles

1 tablespoon fresh cilantro

¼ cup roasted organic corn

1 teaspoon lime juice

Crushed red pepper

½ tablespoon garlic

¼ cup onions

¼ cup black beans

¼ cup hot peppers, or to taste

¼ cup red and orange bell peppers

2 15-ounce cans organic tomatoes

◆ Mix all ingredients together in a large bowl.

JOINT PROTECTION SAUCE

◆ Combine 1 tablespoon finely chopped sautéed garlic, 1 teaspoon cilantro, 1 teaspoon oregano, 1 teaspoon flaxseed oil, ⅓ cup vinegar, ⅓ cup olive oil, and hot sauce to taste.

HUMMUS HIGH

◆ Combine 1 15-ounce can organic chickpeas, mashed; 3 crushed cloves of garlic; juice of ½ lemon; ½ cup finely chopped roasted red bell peppers; and 3 dashes hot sauce.

Hydration

- Purified water
- Glass of purified water with squeezed lemon or lime and a packet of your favorite sweetener
- 100% juice mixed with seltzer water

SNACKS AND PREWORKOUT SNACKS

Snacks

- Jerky: All-natural beef, turkey, ahi tuna, and salmon (my favorite)
- Small bowl of cold tabouli or gazpacho
- Hummus and sliced tomato on half of a whole-wheat pita
- 2 sliced carrots, 1 sliced cucumber, and 3 tablespoons of salsa
- Handful of sunflower seeds
- Bowl of organic popcorn
- Low-fat or nonfat cottage cheese with finely chopped fresh fruit and a sprinkle of organic granola
- 6 ounces of low-fat plain yogurt with berries and sprinkle of organic granola
- Handful of organic raisins, cranberries, pretzels, or 2 organic fig bars with small glass of organic skim milk

Pre-workout Snacks

- ½ of Baker's Breakfast Cookie
- Organic 7-grain toast with a light layer of all-natural organic almond butter

- 8 ounces 100% orange juice
- 6 ounces 100% pomegranate or organic blueberry juice
- Apple with 1 tablespoon all-natural organic peanut butter
- 1 slice whole-grain bread with thinly sliced light cheddar cheese
- 1 banana with 4 ounces organic skim milk
- Handful of almonds with half a piece of organic fruit
- 1 slice of organic hemp sprouted bread with a drizzle of honey

NUTRITION FACTS

Nutrition Label

Breakfast Cookie: Apple Pie

Nutrition Facts	Amount/Serving	% Daily Value*	Amount/Serving	% Daily Value*
Serving Size 1 Cookie (85g) Servings Per Container 1	**Total Fat** 3g	**5%**	**Sodium** 250mg	**10%**
	Saturated Fat 0g	**0%**	**Total Carbohydrate** 55g	**18%**
	Trans Fat 0g		Dietary Fiber 5g	**20%**
Calories 270	**Cholesterol** 0mg	**0%**	Sugars 21g	
Calories from Fat 30			**Protein** 5g	
*Percent Daily Values are based on a 2,000 calorie diet.	Vitamin A 6% • Vitamin C 6%		Calcium 4% • Iron 15%	

Ingredients: Unbleached wheat flour (unbleached wheat flour, niacin, reduced iron, thiamin mononitrate, riboflavin, folic acid), rolled oats, prune puree, organic evaporated cane juice, unsweetened apple sauce, brown rice syrup, dried apples, chicory extract, expeller pressed canola oil, molasses, water, apple pie spice (cinnamon, nutmeg, cloves, cardamom, ginger), natural apple flavor, baking soda, soy lecithin, dried egg whites, cinnamon, aluminum-free baking powder, pure vanilla extract, natural flavor, sea salt.

1. **Serving Size:** This is the first nutrition fact to examine. Many food companies try to fool you by providing an artificially small serving size. You may, for example, take a quick glance at the calorie count *without* looking at the serving size and consume two to three times the serving size. So read the serving size first, before any other nutrition facts.

2. **Calories:** This represents the amount of energy within the food you are consuming. It's an all-important fact to help you realize how much you are consuming during a meal, as well as throughout the day.

3. **Total Fat:** This gives you the collective total of saturated, monounsaturated, polyunsaturated, and trans fats. Not all fats are made equal, far from it, so make sure there are neither trans fats nor much saturated fats (which should be not more than a quarter of total fat consumption). The monounsaturated and polyunsaturated fats—if listed; manufacturers do not have to list these—are the good stuff.

4. **Sodium:** This is salt within the food product. If you have high blood pressure, then pay close attention to this number. Consult your physician on the appropriate levels you are allowed to consume per day.

5. **Total Carbohydrate:** The low-carb diet fad got many people obsessed with this number. Since you are exercising with Hyperstrength, carbohydrates are needed in your daily consumption. Do not pay much attention to this number.

6. **Dietary Fiber:** Eat a diet high in fiber, which benefits both your digestive and circulatory tracts. It is also helps you feel full longer and provides sustaining energy. I try to get at least 3 grams of fiber per serving. The more fiber, the better it is for you.

7. **Sugars:** White sugars and added sugars are bad news—avoid them as much as you can. Worst of all is high fructose corn syrup, so never buy any product with it in the ingredients. Natural sugars, meanwhile, don't need to be fussed about, such as those you find in your fruits, organic milk, and so on.

8. **Protein:** Like carbohydrates, many people have been encouraged to focus on this number as well, sometimes to the detriment of their health. Protein will aid your body when recovering from your Hyperstrength workouts and

keep you feeling full, but most likely your diet is receiving sufficient amounts of protein. You don't need to consume protein-fortified cereals, protein shakes, and a monster-size protein serving at dinner. Instead, follow a simple rule: Try to get quality protein in every meal, whether from dairy, poultry, fish, beef, venison, or another source.

9. **Ingredients:** Always look at the nutritional ingredients you are consuming. If you cannot pronounce the ingredients, chances are those ingredients are processed and bad for your body. Remember, the ingredients are listed in order of the percentage that the product contains, so the first ingredient listed is what the product contains the most of, and so on down the line.

Note: 1) Since you are following the Hyperfare plan, do not worry too much about the rest of the nutritional facts provided. You are getting sufficient vitamins and minerals from the foods you are eating. 2) Many of the foods you will eat, hopefully, will *not* have such labels, because they will be whole, mostly organic produce and meat and dairy from the farmers' market, natural foods store, or even straight from the farm! That being said, these nine nutritional facts are important gauges for any of your everyday foods.

RECOVERY WORKOUTS: BREAK GLASS AND USE WHEN NECESSARY

Pool

1. Side leg lift, 40 reps each side using the side of the pool for support
2. In squat position with your palms out and arms extended, perform squats twisting your midsection left and right, 50 reps
3. In squat position with your arms together, do reverse fly under water while performing squats, 50 reps
4. Freestyle stroke across the pool using your arms only and with your head above water, 8 times
5. Breaststroke across the pool using your arms only and with your head above water, 8 times
6. Swim under water to the other side of the pool, 6 times
7. Place your back against the side of the pool edge, hold the sides, and perform little kicks with your legs, 1 minute, 30 seconds rest, then repeat 5 more times
8. Kickboard variations: Hold in front, hug, straight up, palms on top, and body turned around facing down, then perform little kicks, 3 times for each exercise
9. Shark! Run to Push-up: Run from one end of the shallow end to the other,

jump out of the water, and do push-ups. Start with 40 push-ups, repeat to 30, 20, and 10

10. Squat jump: 50 reps, 50 reps, 60 reps, with 2 big breaths in between sets
11. Lateral hop from one leg to the other, 30 reps each leg

Treadmill

Pick a programmed workout, such as hills. This is a wonderful time to practice your form and proper breathing. Work on higher feet turnover rate, which will make you a faster runner. If your stride falls below 90 strides per minute, practice shortening your stride.

Inline Skating

Find rolling hills and a flat paved surface of at least 4 miles, and practice your stride and gliding like a long-distance speed skater. Set yourself in a relaxed position, then stride and glide in a bent forward stance, with your center of gravity over the skates. With one or both arms behind your back, you will have more efficiency, better balance, and a good power level in your kickoffs. In-line training is a great way to flush out excess lactic acid and give those joints a break. Break up the skating workout by performing sprints and crossovers. Work to marathon distance workouts of 26 miles.

Elliptical Machine

With an elliptical machine, I always add another 1 or 2 exercises to keep me from going stale for the allotted time of the workout. For example: Jump off every 4 to 5 minutes, grab a dumbbell, body bar, or medicine ball, and take to the stairs for 5 times up and down. Then jump back on the elliptical machine for another 4 to 5 minutes, and jump off for push-ups to jump claps above the head for 20 reps. Repeat this series for desired time. It will burn more calories, provide recovery, and help mix up the pace.

Stairclimber Machine

This is one of my favorite health club, nonthinking, zone training pieces of equipment. What's more nonthinking than going up a virtual set of stairs? When my mind does not like placing exercises and programs together, and my body is telling me it needs a little break, I head to this piece of equipment. I usually stick to the pre-programs offered (speed training or fat burn) for the workout.

Cycle: Geared or Single-Speed

One of my favorite workouts for recovery is a single-speed/fixed-gear cycling workout. No gears, no worries, just straight human-powered fun. If there is a hill, you must get out of the saddle to climb it, because you have just one gear. Fixed gear means there is no coasting—your pedals just keep moving. My recovery workout consists in pedaling anywhere and everywhere within a 50 to 75 mile radius from my home. I prefer to cycle when I do my errands. I try not to use my car at all for at least three to four days, and cardio-commute everywhere instead. If you have a place where you need to go, it gives your workout more of a sense of purpose.

Trail Running

Find a park and enjoy the environment as you run through nature. Do not worry about pace, time, distance, heart rate, and so on. Try to listen to every animal and nature sound you can—get in tune with all your senses.

HYPERFITNESS EXERTION SCALE (H.E.S.)

Sector	Exertion Level	Description	Heart Rate Percentages	
1	Low/High	Warming body muscles, light aerobic, recovery workouts, and/or active recovery days off from training	60%	70%
2	Low/High	HyperReal aerobic heart rate (Hyperstrength Base Building)	70%	80%
3*	Low/High	HyperAerobic endurance heart rate (Hyperstrength Endurance Building)	85%	100%
4	Low/High	HyperMax heart rate (Hyperstrength Speed and Muscle Training)	100%	Max
*Between sectors 3 and 4, you reach your AC (Aerobic Ceiling) Heart Rate				

H.E.S. Guide

Begin with your AC Heart Rate, by subtracting your age from 180, and then adjust according to your current fitness lifestyle (below).

- **Trekker:** If you've been exercising inconsistently and you are now in Trekker phase, subtract 5 beats. If you haven't been exercising at all, then subtract 10 beats.

- **Climber:** If you regularly exercise 2 to 3 days a week, keep the number (2 days) or add 5 beats (3 days).
- **Sherpa:** If you work out regularly and consistently at higher than usual levels, add 10 to 15 beats.

Sectors 1–3 Hyperstrength exercises include Base Building, Tempo, and Active Recovery exercises. Sector 4 Hyperstrength exercises include Inner Everest Drills, Speed and Power exercises.

Each person's max varies, regardless of the range they fall into for their age.

H.E.S. Definitions

Resting Heart Rate: Your heart rate at absolute rest.

H.E.S. 1: During warm-ups and a majority of your recovery stage workouts, you will be in this sector. Focus on muscle memory and form performance, balance, and cadence/feet turnover when you're on the bike.

H.E.S. 2: During your zone training and building a solid aerobic base, you will be in sector 2. You will also burn a higher percentage of fat and sugar here.

H.E.S. 3: In this phase, your body learns to tolerate lactic acid buildup while it is training. Hyperstrength was developed to enhance your Sector 3 training to its max. You will also enhance carbohydrate burning and increase fat burn percentage.

H.E.S. 4: You will spend the least amount of time in this sector. There are short bursts within the Hyperstrength workouts that take your body into this range. Too much time within this sector, however, can and will lead to overtraining. If your heart rate spends a large amount of time here on consecutive workouts, swap out a Hyperstrength day for a Recovery Workout.

RMR (Resting Metabolic Rate): Provides the means to calculate the number of calories per day that the body requires.

VO_2: The capacity of the lungs to provide the oxygen that muscles require.

AC: At your aerobic threshold, your muscles become overwhelmed by lactic acid produced by the working muscles. At AC, the amount of CO_2 in your breath dramatically increases and you are no longer able to burn energy efficiently.

Aerobic Endurance: Excellent for increased blood flow, slow-twitch muscle fiber strengthening, heart strengthening, and storing of glycogen in the muscles.

Anaerobic: Anaerobic training enhances fast-twitch muscle fibers, lactate threshold, HR stroke volume, and VO_2 max. This type of training is what can turn a good athlete into a great one.

RESOURCE GUIDE

COMPANY	COMMENTS	WEBSITE
Baker's Wholesome Baked Goods	All-natural, energizing, and healthy products that provide nourishment before, during, and after your Hyperstrength workouts.	bbcookies.com
Burch Hyperfitness Systems LLC	See all the phase levels from the book live— go to the BHS website and order the DVDs.	hyperfitnessliving.com
Fitness Resource	All the equipment you'll need to turn your home gym into a Hyperstrength mecca: Bosu, medicine balls, kettlebells, steps, stability balls, and so on.	fitnessresource.com
Guayakí	The finest organic, rainforest-grown, fairly traded yerba maté on earth, including java maté.	guayaki.com
Hampton	Their Dura-Bells (dumbbells) are top-notch, don't chip, and can take a pounding.	hamptonfit.com
Hoist Equipment	The complete personal cable-training system (PTS) for your home gym.	hoistfitness.com
Hyperfitness Web TV	Web TV for people who want to learn how to live the fitness adventure lifestyle.	hyperfitness.tv
Livity Outernational	Makes functional and stylish products from sustainable materials such as straw, hemp, organic cotton, bamboo, recycled plastic bottles, and veggie-oil-based synthetics.	livity.org
Manitoba Harvest	Provides the freshest and highest-quality hemp food products in the world.	manitobaharvest.com

COMPANY	COMMENTS	WEBSITE
Pacemaster	Quality, commercial-grade treadmills at a consumer-based price; Platinum Pro VR for exceptional decline/incline-based programs.	pacemaster.com
PPC	Provides advanced scientific techniques available for treating the structural problems afflicting the human frame.	perfectposturechiropractic.com
RBH Designs	Custom-designed clothes and mitts for everyday weather as well as the coldest environments around the world.	rbhdesigns.com
Sambazon	Açaí fruit and juice products from the world's #1 source for antioxidant-rich Amazon superfood.	sambazon.com
Amazing Grass	Provides the most potent and convenient way to help achieve your five-plus daily servings of organic fruits and vegetables.	amazinggrass.com
Teko	Recycled, durable, stench-proof, and extremely comfortable socks.	tekosocks.com
World Wildlife Fund	The WWF directs its conservation efforts toward three global goals: saving endangered species, protecting endangered habitats, and addressing global threats such as toxic pollution, overfishing, and climate change.	wwf.org

INDEX